Health promotion
A psychosocial approach

Christine Stephens

Open University Press

Open University Press
McGraw-Hill Education
McGraw-Hill House
Shoppenhangers Road
Maidenhead
Berkshire
England
SL6 2QL

email: enquiries@openup.co.uk
world wide web: www.openup.co.uk

and Two Penn Plaza, New York, NY 10121-2289, USA

First published 2008

A catalogue record of this book is available from the British Library

ISBN–10 0335 22208 0 (pb)   0 335 22209 9 (hb)
ISBN–13 978 0335 22208 7 (pb)   978 0 335 22209 4 (hb)

Library of Congress Cataloging-in-Publication Data
CIP data has been applied for

Typeset by RefineCatch Limited, Bungay, Suffolk
Printed in the UK by Bell and Bain Ltd., Glasgow

The **McGraw-Hill** Companies

Dedicated to Peter Gilbert Lloyd Allen
1923–2005

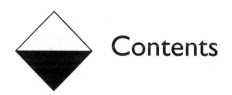

Contents

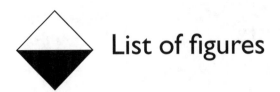

List of figures

Series editors' foreword

This series of books in health psychology has been in progress for over a decade. It is quite remarkable that in so short a period we have seen health psychology change from a marginal topic to a much more mainstream position. This has been a time of rapid growth in the popularity of health psychology as a taught subject at undergraduate and postgraduate level in universities around the world. In addition, health psychology is also emerging strongly as an important 'voice' in psychology with influential things to say about health promotion, health care services and health experiences for those with acute and chronic conditions. Concerned as it is with the application of psychological theories and models to the promotion and maintenance of health and the individual and interpersonal aspects of adaptive behaviour in illness and disability, health psychology has a wide remit. Health psychologists are working in many areas including influencing health care policies at national level, investigating new interventions and health behaviours and working directly with clients or in multidisciplinary teams to deliver good psychological care for those facing illness and impairment. Our book series was designed to support postgraduate and post-qualification studies in psychology, nursing, medicine and paramedical sciences and health psychology units in the undergraduate curriculum.

We are particularly pleased to have Dr Chris Stephens' timely book in the series. In it, she has taken a topical, critical look at planning, implementing and evaluating health promotion. In this view, health is set firmly in its social, economic and political environments. In making her case for the power of these environmental contexts in people's everyday lives, Dr Stephens has taken an international perspective and has drawn on work from other disciplines such as social anthropology, social epidemiology, sociology and community psychology. She has considered anew the research evidence for social determinants of health and the potential role of public policy in shaping the kinds of societies in which health may be promoted for all. In this view of health, risk factors such as smoking and poor diet are seen as symptoms of societal malaise rather than as matters of individual behaviour. Individually based theories of health have produced interventions with disappointing results because they neglect the fact that behaviours are, first and foremost, shaped by the communities in which people are deeply embedded.

Dr Stephens considers the problems with defining the concept of community. For practical reasons, in health promotion 'community' has tended to be defined in terms of geographical location, whereas the communities with which one identifies are likely to be the major influence on health practices. The importance of engaging with and negotiating with these communities in planning, implementing and evaluating health promotion interventions is discussed. Issues around power relationships, partnership and the transfer of power and responsibility to local people are considered. Dr Stephens presents compelling arguments and evidence for effective health promotion to be an essentially community-based, social learning process with active participation by target community groups.

Based on her extensive experience of teaching health promotion to undergraduates and her careful and critical reading of the literature, Dr Stephens has produced an excellent book. She communicates in an engaging and concise style that is likely to be equally appealing to novice students and more experienced researchers. There are many important questions to be answered about health promotion and the role of health psychology; this book sets the stage for new readers. We warmly welcome readers to this challenging and engaging new book.

Sheila Payne and Sandra Horn
Series Editors

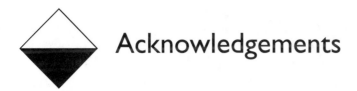

Acknowledgements

The custom of acknowledging the people who have contributed to any work drives home one underlying thesis of this book – that we are embedded in a social world. Although I am named as author of this book, a whole raft of friends and colleagues has supported me and its production. Altogether they are too numerous to name but I am glad to be able to acknowledge all their help, and some particular contributions to this work and its direction. Katy Hamilton, an editorial assistant at McGraw-Hill has been a constant, supportive beacon across the past year. My health psychology colleagues at Massey University, Kerry Chamberlain and Antonia Lyons, have been the most encouraging mentors and friends that one could ask for. Among the rest of the international critical health psychology group I owe special thanks to Wendy Stainton-Rogers, Michael Murray, Catherine Campbell, Uwe Flick, David Marks and Alan Radley. These people have been not only inspirational, but also very generous and hospitable. Christina Lee has been a particularly important part of the process. A woman of fierce intellect and quick wit, she is also the most egalitarian dispenser of support and kindness to all. Christina gave me a space at the University of Queensland and in her home while I was writing some of this book, and also introduced me to many aspects of Australian culture. At home I am fortunate to belong to a very special group of friends, especially Julie and Joanne who have long been rocks of love and care. I am surrounded by caring neighbours, notably Stuart, Olive, Prue, Rod, Toshi and Bruce. I also have a great family and am especially buoyed along in daily life by my husband Robin, my mother Vivienne, my children Jacqueline and Francis, special children Mita and Amelia, our godchildren Ananda and Kiran, and our granddaughter, the beautiful Macy.

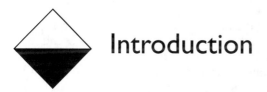# Introduction

The basis of this book was developed as I taught a postgraduate course in health promotion as part of a health psychology programme in New Zealand (also known as Aotearoa). In the early stages, I used traditional psychological theories and research as a basis for suggesting practice in health promotion. However, this basis has been developed across the years and changed quite radically – to fit the needs of my students in actual practice and to align their understandings with current practice in health promotion. One influence was the local context. In New Zealand, health promotion is heavily influenced by a public health model, by the Ottawa Charter and by the Treaty of Waitangi whose principles of bicultural governance, protection of minorities and equal participation guide health related policy. In my work with public health practitioners and advocates, I quickly learned that from this perspective, individual models of health behaviour are seen by many as passé and psychologists trained to implement these models would find it difficult to fit in and share ideas. Another strong influence has been the rapid development of an internationally based critical movement in health psychology. At first, critical health psychologists were concerned to understand health from a social rather than a medically dominated perspective. They drew on work in other disciplines such as sociology and anthropology to develop these understandings. The momentum begun by these changes in research focus and methodology influenced changes in approaches to practice. In health promotion, critical psychologists aligned themselves with community psychologists, public health workers and liberation psychologists to consider the social and structural effects on health, and to call for action toward community-based change and social justice.

These influences have lead to the development and definition of new areas of health psychology such as public health psychology and community health psychology whose approaches to health promotion will be outlined in more detail across the following chapters. Within these approaches, health is understood as an aspect of community life, and an outcome for people in groups and populations. Rather than being the property and responsibility of individuals, health is understood as being related to social, economic and political contexts. From this perspective, there is more emphasis on preventing illness and promoting healthy environments to benefit all. One of the major shifts occasioned by these new influences is that psychological perspectives have become more inclusive and cross-disciplinary. A psychosocial perspective must include understandings of social life and the environmental context of everyday practices. Accordingly, we have needed to draw on information from other disciplines, such as theories of social life from sociology and anthropology, data about the effects of social structure from public health and social epidemiology, and new research methods and practices from areas such as health promotion and community psychology.

The chapters in this book are designed to provide a structured overview of this psychosocial perspective on health promotion. Each chapter deals with a different aspect of health promotion research and practice from choosing health related issues, to examples of interventions and their evaluation. Chapter 1 describes the shift from individually focused theory and practice to a recognition of the fundamentally social nature of health. In this chapter, the implications of this shift for a psychology of health promotion are detailed in terms of moves in health promotion practice. Three major shifts are explained: from a focus on illness to a focus on promoting well being; from aims to change individual behaviour to aims to empower people to be in charge of their own behaviour; and from instrumentally based approaches to ethically based approaches. Chapter 2 discusses the many ways in which a health issue may be chosen as a focus for intervention. The importance of considering this as a choice is discussed, and the value laden and ethical aspects of such choices are brought into the foreground for discussion. Chapter 3 extends this discussion by focusing on one particular health issue: inequalities in health. This chapter details the evidence for the effects of social inequalities on health, and discusses the debates about the meaning of this evidence and the importance of these debates for directing health promotion action on many levels. The wealth of compelling evidence for health inequalities in many societies, and the lack of understanding of the basic cause of the problem, highlights the need for good theories or explanations of health related issues as the basis for health promotion. Thus, Chapter 4 provides an overview of theories that are available to explain health and health behaviours from a social perspective. Chapter 5 follows the discussion of theory with an outline of methods that are available to enquire into health and health related issues. This chapter is structured to emphasize the point that research methods are based on theories, and the methods that we choose are related to the theoretical assumptions that we have about health. Chapter 6 follows the same vein to discuss examples of the theoretical models that are available to guide health promotion practice and intervention. Chapter 7 provides a set of examples of health promotion interventions from a social perspective, conducted at the community level. It is expected that by the time the reader arrives at this chapter, they are equipped to critically evaluate the theoretical basis of these interventions with regard to their purposes and the values inherent in their application. Chapter 8 describes approaches and problems in the evaluation of these sorts of interventions. This chapter follows from the practice examples, but also draws on the readers' understandings of the application of theory, methodology and practice, developed in previous chapters.

Thus, Chapters 1 to 8 may be seen to follow a linear thread: from the development of health promotion practice to include understandings of the social perspective and the choice of health issues through to the subsequent implementation and evaluation of socially based interventions to improve health. However, there are also three main themes running across these chapters and the first is that these choices are iterative, ongoing and circular. Thus, issues are always up for evaluation, and the evaluation of any project must start at the very beginning with the choice of issues and theoretical approach to these issues. All aspects of any project are simultaneously important and all may be constantly being evaluated in various ways.

This recognition leads us to the second major theme, which is reflexivity and values. Although the theoretical assumptions underlying any health promotion activity are often taken for granted, a reflexive approach brings these aspects into the foreground. The importance of reflecting and being able to reflect on all of the choices made across health promotion work is emphasized across the chapters. The reason for highlighting such a reflexive approach is that the theoretical choices that guide our understandings of health also reflect our values. Values themselves deserve to be examined and brought into the light as the basis of certain choices rather than being hidden behind customary practice or utilitarian principles. What is it that we value, and why do we want particular changes? These sorts of questions are raised by a values-based approach which emphasizes the moral nature of health promotion enterprise and the values inherent in every aspect of practice. The shift in values which accompanies a shift to social and community approaches informs the whole book and is mentioned at relevant moments throughout.

The third theme then is the importance of theory and the values inherent in the choice of theoretical approach. Although theory and practice have been seen as a dichotomy since the time of Aristotle, with some practitioners eschewing theory as a sort of navel gazing exercise for academics, all practice is based in theory of some kind. The theory used by many practitioners may simply be unexamined theoretical assumptions. Theory, research and practice lie along a recursive continuum which should be familiar ground to professionals working in any aspect of health promotion. In accord with this understanding, this book gives primacy to all three of these aspects of work in the area of health promotion, which are intimately connected and not easily separated into discrete topics. For example, by beginning with issues and empirical research I have already introduced important aspects of theory, research and practice. However, in the interests of imposing some sort of structure on the book, separate chapters are used to highlight issues regarding theory, methodology and models for practice.

The book is not designed as a definitive guide to any areas of research and practice, but rather as an introduction to the values and assumptions of a socially oriented approach to health promotion, and an invitation to be ongoingly reflexive about our own values and practice. Each chapter ends with some suggestions for further reading, however, the basis of these suggestions varies from chapter to chapter and they should only be taken as suggestions to suit particular interests. The book also provides a number of examples to illustrate the main themes of each chapter, and many of these are excellent works in their own right which I would encourage a reader to follow up. But, even as this book goes to press, new reports are being published in journals, books and on the Internet. Other practitioners are too involved in their practical work to publish and require seeking out through professional connections. It is hoped that the book serves as a spark to encourage further exploration of some of the very exciting and dedicated work in the field of health promotion practice from a social perspective.

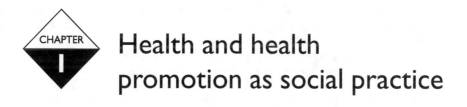

Health and health promotion as social practice

CHAPTER 1

Introduction

In this chapter, I will begin with a discussion around changing notions of health and health promotion, and how these fit with health psychology. The chapter has been organized into three sections to highlight the central themes of social relations, and reflexive research and practice, which will be reiterated throughout the book. The first section addresses understandings of the social location of health. From a social perspective, health is understood as much more than a matter for individual experience and responsibility: health behaviour is seen in terms of relations with others, and health is structured by society. Second, the chapter describes understandings of health promotion as socially and politically constructed. This includes an overview of the history of the changing views of health promotion and the different perspectives and values of health promotion practice. Third, in the light of these understandings, the chapter addresses the changing aims of health promoters and how these changes have affected the ways in which we approach working to improve the health of people in communities and understanding the effects of our own practice.

The social location of health

Health is social

Health concerns in Western societies have been dominated by a biomedical model of health and illness for over 200 years, and the medical perspective dominates our views of health today. This model has also been imposed on other cultures such as those in colonized countries (Durie, 1998). From this perspective, health is located only in the body; a physical entity quite separate from psychological and social processes. The development of behavioural approaches to medicine, and health psychology as a discipline, has included the importance of the mind to illness and well being (Lyons and Chamberlain, 2006). Psychology is a discipline focused on the individual as the basis of thought and behaviour, and this individual approach has mapped very well onto the medical model of the mechanical body. The well known 'biopsychosocial model' of health (Engel, 1977) introduced a more holistic approach to explaining health. However, the ways in which mind, body and social life work actually together have not been well conceptualized or developed since, and the model has remained an ideal image, rather than providing guidance for understanding.

From the biomedical perspective, epidemiological work has shown that groups within populations, such as those of gender, ethnicity, socioeconomic status and age, have marked and reliable differences in health. Many of these have been explained in terms of physiological differences, such as deterioration with age or genetic weaknesses in certain groups. However, there is increasing evidence to show that many of the regular differences cannot be explained biologically. For example, why do women live longer than men these days, and yet women generally have more illness than men? Some answers come from large bodies of work in psychology and epidemiology, which demonstrate strong and reliable relationships between constructs such as social support or social networks and health (Seeman, 1996; Berkman et al., 2000). In addition, a great deal of evidence about the importance of social life can be found in research from other disciplines such as sociological and anthropological inquiry which has pointed to the very social nature of categories such as gender and age. Critical enquiries have shown both the impact of social life on well being, and the socialized nature of research and treatment itself which leads to observed differences. For example, women are more likely to experience ill health and also less likely to receive diagnoses and treatment for illnesses such as heart disease (Rodin and Ickovics, 1990; Annandale and Hunt, 2000). Members of oppressed minority groups, who are more likely to suffer ill health and early death, are also subject to discrimination in everyday life and in access to health care services (Smedley et al., 2003; Blakely et al., 2006). A growing body of interpretive work has shown that people hold diverse, culturally and socially bound understandings of the meanings of health, suffering, disease and behaviours that might affect health (Radley, 1993; Hardey, 1998; Levin and Browner, 2005).

Health behaviour is relational

Health related behaviour has been seen as underlying many modern ills such as cancer, heart disease, infectious diseases and the outcomes of many chronic diseases. Many health promoters feel that if people could be persuaded to eat healthy foods, engage in exercise, safe sex and other safety practices, screen their bodies for disease and manage their stress, then they would be healthier. It turns out that there are some problems with this apparently simple plan, and many of them may be explained by the lack of understanding of the very social nature of behaviour. For example, we do not necessarily do things with a disease outcome in mind. There are many socially located explanations for our behaviour that we are not even necessarily aware of as individuals. Some behaviours only make sense in certain social contexts or have different meanings within different relationships. In addition, there are many layers and forces in any society. Requirements to conform with ideals, mores and moral strictures, from family, peers and wider society, are far more important to our social well being than the requirement to prevent disease. Moreover, many of us are controlled by others with greater power and more access to resources. Our ideal health related behaviour and a healthy environment are not necessarily within our own control. In sum, the fundamental importance of social life to everyday being in the world means that any actions that impact on our health are much more than the result of an individual decision to act in a certain way.

Crossley (2000a) provides some provocative examples of the ways in which our social life is entwined with the things we do. Qualitative enquiries cited by Crossley show young mothers using smoking as a positive resource within daily struggles against pressures and lack of support, or risky behaviours such as unprotected sex are seen by young men as a symbolic assertion of living a full life. Ironically, it is the very strictures suggested by health promotion that provide the basis for such rebellion.

Qualitative enquiry has shown that social relationships do not just shape or influence health behaviours. Rather, the shared language of participants in particular contexts constructs particular actions as being meaningful in specific ways. For example, using a condom in a classroom has a completely different meaning to its use in sexual intercourse. Thus, an individual may quite honestly report an intention to act in a certain way that is inconsistent with later actions. Willig (1999) has analysed people's talk about condom use in relationships to show how meanings such as trust and romance (not just protection) are an important part of condom use in practice.

The social and structural basis of health

Research into health disparities among population groups has demonstrated that social and economic forces influence health through more than individual health behaviours and individual coping skills; more broadly based psychosocial and environmental risk factors are at work (Smedley, 2006). The relationship between social inequalities and health was highlighted by the British Black Report (Townsend and Davidson, 1982). This report highlighted a great deal of evidence for inequalities in health between social groups, and disparities in resources and service provision. The report awakened a surge of international research in health disparities of every sort, to reveal alarming and growing inequalities in health within and between countries.

A renaissance of health inequalities research (Labonte et al., 2005) has lead in turn to a focus on the socially based influences on health. In 1998, WHO published *The Social Determinants of Health: The Solid Facts*, which has since been updated in a second edition (Wilkinson and Marmot, 2003). This publication presents a collection of research evidence for the social determinants of health in the areas of the social gradient, stress, early life, social exclusion, work, unemployment, social support, addiction, food and transport. For each aspect the book suggests the role that public policy can play in shaping a social environment that will support better health.

An important shift in research and policy that has accompanied this new focus is understandings of health as a population issue. Epidemiologists and sociologists have noted that populations have characteristic disease rates or health issues that have causes which cannot be explained by studying individual differences. The implication is that societal interventions may be more effective than targeting individual behaviours, even for behaviours that are traditionally understood and treated as located in personal behaviour such as heavy alcohol consumption (Marmot, 1999).

These understandings have led towards a shift away from an exclusive focus on individually based theories of health behaviour and the need to include conceptions of social life in social policy and health promotion. In 2003, Prilleltensky and Prillelltensky made strong suggestions for critical health psychology practice. They pointed to the disappointing results of individually focused interventions to suggest that 'risk factors' such as diet, smoking and exercise are symptoms of deeper social causes of ill health. One of the effects of this shift has been to start thinking of people as embedded in social groups or communities.

Towards community approaches to health

Whaley (2003) notes that 'the public health approach of individual risk factor modification has proved to be expensive but not very successful' (p. 740). A growing recognition of the shortcomings of individually focused approaches to health promotion, in conjunction with recognition of the importance of social life, has led to the development of new approaches and a focus on people within broader social contexts. One useful descriptive word for this approach is 'community', encapsulating the new focus on groups of people. Community-based approaches to health promotion to address the failures of individual behaviour oriented approaches have become increasingly common since the mid-1970s (Guldan, 1996). However, this shift has been a matter of slow and faltering development rather than transformation. There are many practical, political and institutional issues involved in the moves toward community approaches noted by commentators like Guldan. An issue underlying all of these problems is our understandings of social life and health and meanings of community. It has not been sufficient to transfer individual-based theorizing into community applications and this is still a problem. Commentators still note that the application of individual theories at population levels has proved to be awkward (Hepworth, 2004) and dangerously unethical (Mabala, 2006).

A first step in recognizing the importance of social life has been to consider the cultural context and human relationships as additional factors affecting individuals and their behaviours. However, to understand groups of people as 'organisms' we needed to shift toward understandings of the person as inextricable from their social context: the individual as a part of, product of and producer of that context. Public health workers and health psychologists (whose disciplines are traditionally individually focused) have needed to make some important shifts in their understandings of health and behaviour, and in doing so have called upon explanations and methods from several other disciplines.

Multidisciplinary approaches to public health issues and health promotion have introduced a raft of socially focused theorizing and application from other areas such as community psychology, community development, sociology, social epidemiology, health geography, anthropology, social work, political science and public policy. Many health research groups are deliberately multidisciplinary and interdisciplinary. An example is the Institute of Population Health in Ottawa, Canada, described by Labonte et al. (2005). This centre aims to effect social change based on three central tenets:

1 Health is seen as embedded in social relations of power and historically inscribed contexts.
2 Research should be shaped by the interests of those communities who carry the greatest burden of disease.
3 Research methods should engage community constituencies as active agents in the process of research.

Thus, a focus on the social nature of health has been translated into a focus on communities, including communities of need and communities of power. However, the use of the word 'community' to denote social life has led to some anomalies and issues itself that must be noted here.

'Community' is a word that is used quite freely and often unreflexively in the literature. Goodwin (2003, p. 29) noted that: 'wherever social relations are described, analysed, remembered, or even mythologised, various conceptions of "community" are almost invariably deployed'. Owing to the everyday meaning of the word, and varying conceptions deployed in the literature, community has proved impossible to define consistently. In 1955, Hillery identified 94 different definitions of community in the academic literature on which there is no clear agreement, a situation which has not been resolved by academics to date. For practical purposes, McLeroy et al. (2003) identify four types of community-based interventions: community as the setting; community as the target for change; community as the resource and community as agent. At the same time these authors note that there are many other typologies of community approaches that have been proposed in the literature. Campbell and Murray (2004) describe the focus in the community health arena as being on either communities of identity (such as the 'gay community' or the 'Jewish community') or communities of place (such as neighbourhoods and rural towns). Geographically based communities are most often the target of health promotion work for very pragmatic reasons: areas such as neighbourhoods or towns provide for identification of deprivation and a focal point for gathering people together for community action.

'Community' as a word has positive, friendly connotations and it is often used to strike a positive note in a way that has also been exploited by politicians. In the 1980s and 1990s there were several critiques of the contradictory uses of the notion of community. For example, Bryson and Mowbray (1981) from Australia, called 'community' a 'spray-on solution' to describe the way in which the label had been seized upon and applied in a simplistic way to complex social problems. In 1994, Farrant pointed to gaps between such rhetoric and the reality in UK practice, including issues such as the structural and institutional barriers to actual implementation of community-based development for health. These criticisms have not abated. More recently, Pearce (2003) pointed to the dangers of unexamined assumptions about community as locality in health promotion practice. In a paper entitled, 'Which community?' he raised some practical problems: not all social identities (such as ethnicity or sexual orientation) are geographically based; social networks are more often built through other connections such as work or family; and deprived people do not necessarily live in deprived areas. Pearce's underlying critique is that targeting resources and power to local areas can lead to the suppression of minority groups in these areas, whereas more centrally devolved provision can provide for all groups.

Towards developing a coherent theoretical approach for community health work Campbell and Jovchelovitch (2000) defined community in terms of three key dimensions: shared identity; a shared set of social representations; and shared conditions and constraints in access to power. In regard to shared representations, Stephens (2007) has used people's everyday talk about community to show that people have access to multiple social representations of community and these are used to serve different purposes at different times. Thus, health promoters' uses of representations of community are also likely to be deployed contingently. Rather than attempt to hammer out final definitions, it is best to be aware of our use of the word and the purposes that it is serving at any time. In this book, the word 'community' will be used in accord with different theoretical and practical contexts. Thus its use, although not overtly contradictory, may shift across the chapters and we must keep interrogating the social purposes of its application in these different contexts.

Health promotion is socially constructed

Just as health is a part of social life, health promotion as an activity engaged in by people, is socially constructed and a matter for political struggles. One way of understanding this is to look briefly at the history of health promotion and to note the ways in which shifting discourses have been used by health practitioners and politicians to construct health promotion activities.

What is 'health promotion'?

Health promotion involving professionals and organizations is generally sponsored by governments or non-governmental organizations (NGOs) with public good goals. Government funded health promotion in Western countries is usually organized as part of the 'public health' sector of government concern. However, 'public health', as a branch of medicine, is also a discipline in its own right, and these related but different versions of the phrase both signal the dominance of medicine in the field and lead to confusion in the jostling for control of public funding among disciplines and institutions. Webster and French (2003) outline a history of some of the conflicts between public health and health promotion goals while also noting their common interests:

> The goals of public health are usually stated to be 'preventing disease and promoting health' and the mechanisms for realizing these objectives are to be organized interventions directed at particular groups or the community as a whole. Clearly, therefore, public health has always been associated in some way with health promotion
>
> (2003, p. 10)

Shifting constructions of health promotion

There have been major changes in the construction of 'health promotion'. It must be noted that these understandings and ways of talking about promoting health are available and co-exist in practice today. As some come to prominence or new understandings arise, there are ongoing disputes regarding the history and goals of public health activities. Here I will describe some major changes in dominant constructions of health promotion in Western societies to illustrate the shifting nature of understandings of health and health promotion.

Sanitation, health services and health care

In nineteenth century Europe, the early public health movement focused largely on sanitary conditions and especially on housing, water, disposal of waste and working conditions (Webster and French, 2003). These remain important aspects of public health concern in many countries to this day. However, in the twentieth century the emphasis in countries like the UK shifted to a focus on clinics and services, including health education, to deal with the needs of vulnerable groups. Following World War II, this emphasis in many Western countries shifted to the provision of health care services such as GPs, nurses, dentists and hospitals. In other words, to a biomedically dominated approach that valued medical treatment as the focus of public health. In more welfare oriented countries such as the UK and Canada this was the time for the development of extensive state provision of health care which dominated the public health scene.

To those of us who grew up in this era, the provision of medical services does seem to be the fundamental basis of health. The provision of hospitals and access to medical services including general practitioner care and surgical operations are the basis of political competition for votes in countries with state provided services, and the basis of activism and protest in those without. Nevertheless, there have been many critiques of the dominance of biomedical discourses in our understandings of health. Among the famous and influential works are Illich's (1977) *Limits to Medicine: Medical Nemesis, the Expropriation of Health*, whose title is a good indication of content. Another very influential work was McKeown's (1979) *The Role of Medicine* which argued (convincingly for many) that medical care had little to do with the improvements in life expectancy in the UK at the end of the last century.

Lifestyle and health behaviours

A major shift in the way public health was understood took place in the 1970s. Robertson (1998) describes these changes in terms of a change from the dominance of a medical discourse of health to discourses privileging 'health promotion'. There are two important stages in these changes and the discourses that underpin them can be found in two influential documents. First, the Lalonde report (*New Perspectives on the Health of Canadians*) was published in 1974. The Lalonde report introduced the 'health field' concept as an explanatory model including various factors such as lifestyle and environment as determinants of health. Medical health care was positioned as only one of many determinants. The lifestyle aspect of this model dominated health promotion discourse, and individual level behaviour change became a major focus for improving health in the 1970s and 1980s (Robertson, 1998).

There has been a great deal of critique of the effects of this shift. In 1993, Becker who, as a medical sociologist contributed to the health promotion movement and developed a model of health beliefs, also noted what he termed the 'dark sides' of health promotion activities at the end of his career. First, he criticized constant exhortations to the public to change their behaviours, based on cavalier and premature use of tentative research evidence. Thus we see the familiar reversals and contradictions in public health messages that continue today: 'Don't eat eggs, they have bad choles-terol', 'Do eat eggs, they are full of Omega-3'; 'Protect yourself from the sun, it causes cancer', 'Get more sun to avoid vitamin D shortage'. Becker believed that the promises of longer life based on such ill founded messages are unethical. Second, he believed that the relentless nature of such health promotion messages has caused an 'epidemic of apprehension' so that people are needlessly and excessively anxious about the health effects of their behaviours such as their diet. Third, he criticized the tendency of lifestyle health promotion to locate the responsibility for all health issues with the individual. Becker believed that this last issue was the most serious, and many other commentators have pointed to the damaging effects of this shift to individual responsibility. From a cultural and sociological perspec-tive, Petersen and Lupton (1996) suggest that the focus of the new public health on psychological, social and physical aspects of health is, at its core, a moral issue that deserves scrutiny. This scrutiny has been provided by several other commentators who have written about the rise of 'healthism' and the individualization of health concerns. The term 'healthism' was coined by Crawford in 1980 to describe the effect in society of individually focused prevention messages. The emphasis on an individual's obligation to be con-cerned with health and to live a controlled life, valuing self-restraint and avoidance of risk, has lead to a moral climate in which people feel they have failed if they do contract disease; people may be blamed for their own illnesses; and some may be denied health care for diseases linked to 'bad' behaviours.

Social determinants and empowerment

The dominance of the health fields model in health promotion was extended by a second major influential document. The Ottawa Charter for Health Promotion (1986) which built on concepts of health from the WHO's Global Strategy for Health for All by the Year 2000 (1981). These publications redefined health as broad-based well being rather than just the absence of disease. Based on growing evidence for the social determinants of health, they included factors such as poverty, social exclusion, unemploy-ment and poor housing as providing the basis of health outcomes. These reports also suggested new focuses and methodologies for health promotion. A new focus on public policy and cooperation between government sectors such as housing, transport and health was called for. New methodologies such as community development, empowerment of people to take charge of their own health, advocacy and social marketing were promoted. The result-ing radical shift to policies and approaches based on social explanations of health, including the importance of social interaction and participation as important aspects of well being, became known as 'health promotion' or 'the new public health'.

Of course, the dominance of particular constructions of the purposes and methods of health practice do not stand still. There are ongoing shifts, jostling for economic and ideogical prominence, and related discussions in the literature about the choices and policies of successive governments, public health officials and institutions. For example, in her critique of shifting discourses, Robertson (1998) criticized the increasingly popular notion of 'population health' in public health discourse. In contrast to health promotion, she describes this approach as devoid of theory or concerns for morality and social justice, and denying the political aspects of health practice. Porter (2007) has followed these lines to critique the 2005 WHO Bangkok Charter for Health Promotion in a Globalised World. She compares the discourses used in this report with the Ottawa Charter of 1986 and notes a shift from a 'new social movements' discourse of environmental and social justice to a 'new capitalist' discourse focused on law and economics. Porter compares this new discourse with that of economic determinants promoted by the population health approach. Labonte also 'lamented the rise of the "population health" discourse' in 1997. However, later (Labonte et al., 2005) he describes the development of a critical approach to population health research which can include theoretical engagement and social and moral values.

The practice of health promotion

As the discourses of public health impact directly on people's understandings of their health and lifestyles, so these shifting discourses construct the practice of health promoters. In 2005, Fairhurst noted that health promotion and community health workers were now expected to respond to calls for a social model of health embracing environmental matters, active participation by members of the public, and recognition of the importance of the structure of communities and society. Thus, health promotion professionals must respond as social policy and organizational demands change. These responses have lead to some notable shifts in health promotion practice: from a focus on pathology to a focus on well being; from aims of behaviour change to aims of empowerment and participation; and from the choice of instrumentally based approaches to ethically based choices.

From pathology to well being

In 1948 the WHO reconceptualized health as a positive state with their famous definition which has not been amended since (WHO, 2008): 'Health is a state of complete physical, mental and social well-being and not merely the absence of disease or infirmity.' (This was the preamble to the Constitution of the World Health Organization as adopted by the International Health Conference, New York, 19 June–22 July 1946; signed on 22 July 1946 by the representatives of 61 States (Official Records of World Health Organization, no. 2, p. 100) and entered into force on 7 1948.) Although this classic definition has proved difficult to conceptualize (Levin and Browner, 2005) and very difficult to operationalize (Saracci, 1997), its symbolic weight signalled the beginning of a renewed understanding that illness and disease are only a small aspect of health. This definition has been an important basis for the aims of health promotion which have increasingly included the social and positive aspects of well being.

Antonovsky (1996) saw that the revolutionary ideas of the new health promotion were in danger of stagnating for lack of coherent theory. He was concerned to develop theory that would enable health promotion to move towards promoting health. In proposing a model for health promotion that would move populations toward better health, Antonovsky developed the notion of 'salutogenesis', a neologism which he had coined in 1979. A 'salutogenic' theory of health rejected the pathogenic orientation of 'all Western medical thinking' which focuses attention on disease and ignores broader interests in well being. Although ignored for many years, Antonovsky's ideas have attracted renewed interest since the 1990s; this interest has centred on the importance of the salutogenic focus in many areas of health promotion practice. For example, Sidell (2003) describes how Antonovsky's framework may be applied to understanding the differences between older people's accounts of their health and morbidity data. This perspective includes health seen as a continuum, rather than as the absence of disease, and provides a new view of health promotion for elders. The aim of helping older people move toward the healthy end of the continuum includes perceptions of the role of ageing unfriendly physical environments and ageist social environments. McCreanor and Watson (2004) similarly use this broader framework to consider the role of physical and social environments in promoting the well being of young people.

The changes in health promotion aims, from those of prevention of sickness to those of promotion of wellness are reflected in the Ottawa Charter for Health Promotion (1986). These have been increasingly drawn upon in the new health promotion movements.

From behaviour change to social change

Recognition of the social location of health has also lead to a shift in the aims of health promotion from individual behaviour change to changes in social conditions that affect health, especially the health of disadvantaged people. In turn, this has brought theories of empowerment and the participation of community members in health promotion activity to the foreground. Thus, there has been a growing focus on 'community' since the new public health developments in the 1970s which draws on conceptualizations from areas such as community development and community psychology, although health psychology has been slow to include these changes.

In the last 20 years there have been some moves toward including a public health orientation and community approaches within health psychology practice. Hepworth (2004) outlined a conceptual and practical framework for a 'public health psychology'. The defining features of practice include 'a focus on public rather than individual health, inequalities in health, multi-method design and multidisciplinary and interdisciplinary practice' (2004, p. 52). In the same issue, Murphy and Bennett (2004) suggested that psychologists adopt a more holistic approach to health. One avenue of this public health oriented approach would be to draw upon the 'long-standing tradition in public health of community involvement' (2004, p. 22). They point to the usefulness of concepts used in these approaches such as empowerment and participation. Nelson et al. (2004) and Murray et al. (2004) consider these shifts as the development of a 'community health psychology'. Community health psychology is characterized by these authors as taking a broader view of health and well being to include the social environment, power inequalities and an ecological perspective in which people are seen as being embedded in small groups which are part of larger systems. Community health psychology interventions strive to change the social conditions that affect health. Rather than be driven by 'experts' who know what changes should be made, a community health psychology emphasizes community driven approaches involving partnerships between professional and community groups.

Campbell (2003), a social psychologist working in health promotion, has summarized the arguments for the importance of community participation in improving health. These include the importance of involving community groups in decisions about health care and in the design of promotion campaigns. In addition, there is the recognition of the environmental and social community conditions on health so that concepts such as community cohesion and empowerment become a focus of activity. Campbell also notes that much remains to be understood about how participation relates to health and although practical application is growing, theoretical understanding is weak. Other critiques of the use of communitarian approaches are noted above.

Rather than focusing solely on the community level of action, a community health psychology also recognizes the importance of wider social systems to the well being of smaller or disadvantaged groups in society. It may include concerns with the broader social context of inequalities and focus efforts toward influencing social policy and working towards social justice. Prilleltensky and Prillelltensky (2003), suggest that engaging in health promotion activities at any level of practice, individual, group or community, must include a critical perspective that challenges the hegemonies and power relations that are apparent within a societal and economic view of health. In particular, they consider the importance of power differences and the effects of inequalities and oppression that are obscured in individualist approaches. Murray and Poland (2006) propose that moving toward a critical health psychology approach to practice includes social action that contributes to the movement for social justice. They suggest that such actions include research that reveals the deleterious impact of unjust social arrangements, advocacy efforts to highlight unhealthy living and working conditions, and engaging in community and collective action to transform unhealthy living conditions. These actions involve connecting with community and liberation psychologists and others who have been engaged in movements for social justice.

From instrumental to ethical

In taking their more radical positions, both Prilleltensky and Prillelltensky (2003) and Murray and Poland (2006) note the importance of an awareness of one's own social position and how this frames our view of the world. This awareness includes becoming sensitive to the values involved in our own theories about health, and the research questions and practical applications that they underpin. It has also supported a shift from an instrumental or strategic approach (which ignores underlying assumptions and values) to a values-based approach to choices about health promotion.

Prilleltensky and Prillelltensky (2003) critique the functionalist or strategic approaches of traditional health psychology and the assumption of scientific neutrality in health promotion practice. Crossley (2001) also critiques the functionalist or strategic approach of traditional health psychology in which the aim is prediction and control of health related behaviour, based on assumptions that researchers and practitioners are objective scientists with privileged access to a body of validated knowledge. The aim to identify and manipulate the predictors of individuals' unhealthy behaviour excludes consideration of values, morality and the reflexive consideration of the practitioners' own values and the values of those they serve in these activities. Stam (2000) also notes that health and health care is a social activity in itself. Focusing on 'individual actors usually obfuscates the complex moral/power relations involved' (p. 274). Thus, there are both moral (What worth do such goals have?) and political (Whose ends do they serve?) questions which are not engaged with in instrumental, individually oriented approaches. Both Prillelltensky and Prilleltensky (2003) and Crossley (2001) draw on critical theorists to argue that instrumental approaches that exclude a recognition of social values support the individualistic ideologies which actively work against the achievement of values of social justice, participation, caring and health.

Seedhouse (1997) argues that ethics is all-pervading in health promotion. Health promotion is a moral endeavour and yet health promoters act as though they are in an ethical vacuum. Seedhouse claims that the perception that health promotion is driven by evidence, and strategies chosen to deal with preventable problems, is simply erroneous. Health promotion is always driven by values, and the evidence and strategies are then selected according to the particular values and political philosophies. Once we acknowledge this, and examine our own values, then we can move forward to acknowledge and discuss the 'political tap roots' of health promotion. To contribute to this shift from an instrumental approach to acknowledging the values behind all choices, Guttman (2000) discusses the ethical dilemmas in health promotion. In her book she has provided cogent analysis and structured suggestions for the ways in which practitioners may shift from strategic analytic approaches to a values-based approach to public health interventions.

Murray et al. (2004) discuss the specific aims and values of a community health psychology. A first aim is seen as the need to broaden our understandings of health and illness to include the social, cultural and political dimensions of health. This has implications for our understandings of the basis of knowledge and the theoretical basis of our research. A second aim is to contribute to a reduction in human suffering and improvement in quality of life. This aim leads to a reconsideration of the role of the practitioner (from detached observer to personal commitment) and the basis of practice. Underlying these changes in approach is a set of acknowledged values. Community health psychologists would value health promotion, the empowerment of oppressed people, action for social justice, diversity, caring, compassion and community.

As the chapters of this book unfold sometimes my own values will be clear with regard to the ways in which we understand health, the different theoretical approaches to health, and the values that we can bring to health promotion activities. However, I have also attempted to provide a reasonably even handed overview of different approaches, theories and methodologies, and so I will clarify my own position here, beginning with a little background. I began my career in health psychology, researching the effects of social support on the experience of post-traumatic stress disorder from a traditional positivist perspective. At the same time I was introduced to critical social psychology, and began a parallel line of study employing discourse analysis. This developed into research on the social basis of women's health issues, followed by research into social connections and how these relate to health. Some time in the middle of this, I began teaching health promotion to graduate students as part of a health psychology course. At the start, I drew on traditional approaches in psychology, such as social cognitive models, and traditional texts, to talk with my students about health and health promotion. Encouraged by discussions with students and practitioners, my own background in critical psychology, and increasing exposure to the work of psychologists such as Michael Murray and Catherine Campbell who were developing community approaches, I included fewer and fewer of the cognitive oriented approaches until they have dropped from my course altogether. They do not fit with my own understandings of the social basis of health and with my values of social justice. Nevertheless, I believe they deserve inclusion in this text owing to their widespread use in psychological research and practice today. As exemplified by my own rather mixed background, the approach towards the focus on social and community approaches that is being suggested by different commentators and practitioners at present has developed from an often ill fitting and confusing range of sources. Rather than deciding what the one right approach is in a prescriptive sort of way, I hope that the overview in this text will work towards enabling us to evaluate all the tools and methods available to us in terms of their implicit values and the values with which we wish to align ourselves. I believe that a community-based approach to health promotion is emerging but will naturally continue to evolve and change as we develop our abilities to critique our own activities on the basis of shared values. Of course, those values themselves are vigorously debated in the literature today. One thing that I would hope that any reader of this text will gain is encouragement to develop a reflexive approach to practice, and the confidence to critically contribute to these debates.

Summary

This chapter has highlighted three important shifts from traditional views of health and health promotion. First, a shift from an understanding of health that has been dominated by the biomedical view of health as a matter for individual bodies and a psychological perspective that sees health as a matter for individual minds. Looking out from under this single-minded view, we are beginning to understand the very social nature of health; that health is a matter for people embedded in social life; that health related behaviour is more about that social life than about health; and that the structure of society contributes to the well being of its members. From this perspective we can understand that health promotion itself is socially constructed. Second, there has been a move from viewing health as a problem – a pathology-based approach – towards a positive view of health. Public health workers who are focused on wellness work are working toward health promotion for all, rather than on disease prevention as an end in itself. The focus on well being fits well with social understandings of health because a great deal of our well being is about social relationships. The third important shift has been moves by health promoters from scientific paradigms, that emphasize prediction and control, towards a concern with meaning and values. This move leads the health promoter away from a role as an expert impartial observer, towards respect for the importance of participation by those whose health needs to improve.

The development and application of these aspects of health promotion, along with the need for a reflexive health promotion practice, will be discussed and illustrated across the following chapters. I will consider them in terms of framing health issues, theoretical and ethical understandings of those issues, theoretical tools available for health promotion research and practice from community perspectives, and examples of community oriented health promotion practice. To begin at the beginning of a process of health promotion intervention, the next chapter will discuss the health issues that we think require some action, and the ways they are chosen.

Further reading

1 An edited collection which focuses on the social determinants of health inequalities including a range of aspects such as socioeconomic status, family, culture, ethnicity, and the physical and political environment:
  Eckersly, R., Dixon, J. and Douglas, B. (eds) (2001) *The Social Origins of Health and Well-being*. Cambridge: Cambridge University Press.
2 A book providing a systematic account of the ways in which health is embedded in the social world, it covers the role of medicine, lay understandings of health, the roles of health services and professionals, and the effects of social class and gender:
  Hardey, M. (1998) *The Social Context of Health*. Buckingham: Open University Press.
3 This paper serves as an introduction to a special issue devoted to a wide variety of anthropological explorations of the social production of health:
  Levin, B.W. and Browner, C.H. (2005) The social production of health: critical contributions form evolutionary, biological, and cultural anthropology, *Social Science & Medicine*, 61, 745–50.
4 Lupton critically examines the new public health to discuss the implications of health promotion practices for people's understandings of risk, their bodies and the use of mass media to regulate populations:
  Lupton, D. (1995) *The Imperative of Health: Public Health and the Regulated Body*. London: Sage.
5 This is a collection of contributions that provide excellent examples of the ways in which illness and health are part of social life and their experience informed by the social world:
  Radley, A. (1993) *Worlds of Illness: Biographical and Cultural Perspectives on Health and Disease*. London: Routledge.

CHAPTER 2

Issues in health promotion

Introduction

A focus on exercise promotion or smoking cessation is often taken for granted by health workers. Sometimes the official focus of a health promotion intervention may be at odds with the primary concerns of the people concerned. For example, health promoters running a community programme to enhance exercise participation found that the main health concerns of the community members were actually related to domestic violence. Thus, the reasons and methods for choosing health issues is an often neglected but important stage to consider in planning research and intervention. In this chapter, I consider how and why particular issues are chosen by health promoters as the basis for their work and what strategies may be employed in these choices. The chapter begins by considering how the evidence for any aspect of health as a concern is selected, the possible sources of evidence for these health concerns, and how theoretical approaches determine the collection and interpretation of evidence. It outlines the different settings and levels (from individual to public policy levels) which provide different foci for health concerns. Finally, the choices are considered in terms of values at every level. The values of stakeholders, researchers and health promoters are embedded in all choices about health issues. This section highlights the importance of examining the values that affect these choices and then the ethical issues that arise from these sorts of considerations.

Evidence for health issues

Given that the fundamental aims and philosophies of health promotion are a moveable feast, how are the actual issues of focus chosen? What are the health issues that practitioners take on as requiring attention and change in some way? David Seedhouse (1997) describes the way that he and his colleagues as health promotion workers in 1986 chose what to do on very practical grounds: 'they were good at something, the health authority desired a particular project, they could be effective, it was a useful experience, clients wanted it' (1997, p. viii). These reasons may be familiar to many local health promoters 30 years later. Some emphases have changed; exercise and diet have become more central issues for health authorities, and the theoretical models of health promotion drawn on by health workers have grown more socially or community oriented. However, smoking and drug use remain major concerns, and many of the strategies used for everyday practice (community classes, information pamphlets) remain largely the same. But what are the bases of these health related concerns?

Nutbeam (1998) draws on the Ottawa Charter to define health promotion in terms of enabling people to improve their health by controlling the determinants of health. The determinants of health include those within the immediate control of individuals, such as individual health behaviours, and those outside individual control, such as social, economic and environmental conditions. How do health promoters decide which determinants are important?

Epidemiological data

Nutbeam suggests two main sources of information for the definition of health issues as the basis for intervention. One is published epidemiological research, which identifies the causes and scope of health problems on a population basis. Whaley (2003) has also observed that epidemiological research has a key role in identifying the important issues that form the basis of health policy and intervention. Two well known examples of how this sort of evidence has been hugely influential are in evidence for the relationship between tobacco smoking and lung disease, and the effects of smoking and diet on coronary heart disease (CHD). Large scale population studies have been used to establish that there is a reliable relationship (although not always uncontentious or unequivocal) between behaviours such as smoking and health outcomes such as lung cancer or other respiratory illnesses. Such population studies may range from public health surveillance data which monitor the prevalence of particular diseases through academic and publicly funded research, to international research projects funded by bodies such as the World Health Organization (WHO).

The World Health Report (WHO, 2002) is one example of an influential document which provides evidence as the basis for focusing on particular health issues. This report included a summary of the major 'risk factors' for reduced health outcomes expressed as total disability adjusted life years

(DALYs: a measure of mortality that takes into account quality of life). The 2002 report describes the amount of disease, disability and death in the world attributable to some of the most important risks to human health. It also shows how much this burden could be lowered in the next 20 years if the same risk factors were reduced. Some examples of the risk factors described in this way are:

Underweight	Cholesterol	Indoor smoke
Iron deficiency	Blood pressure	Lead exposure
Vitamin A	Overweight	Climate change
deficiency	Low fruit and vegetable	Unsafe sex
Zinc deficiency	intake	Lack of contraception
Tobacco	Physical inactivity	Occupational risks
Alcohol	Unsafe water	Injury
Illicit drugs	Air pollution	Ergonomic stressors

The report presents the factors in relation to different countries and it is clear that some risk factors are more likely to be those associated with poor countries (underweight) while others are issues for wealthy countries (overweight). Although the report presents the factors as individual factors many may also be seen in direct relation to one another. For example, poor diet and physical inactivity are associated with obesity, which in turn is associated with high blood pressure.

The focus on 'risk factors' is one way in which the determinants of population health may be understood. An outline of the evidence for different risk factors ignores the social context of health, and an alternative socially oriented view of determinants is presented in *The Solid Facts: Social Determinants of Health* (Wilkinson and Marmot, 2006), a booklet also published by WHO. This publication draws on evidence of inequalities in health within countries and for the importance of the social environment to health. This publication explains how psychological and social influences affect physical health and mortality. It provides evidence for the most important social determinants of health today. Key research sources are given to support the importance to health of stress, early life, social exclusion, working conditions, unemployment, social support, addiction, healthy food and transport policy.

Needs assessment

The second source of information highlighted by Nutbeam is community needs assessment which is used 'to identify community concerns and priorities, to identify access points to reach and work with key individuals, and to enable more direct community participation in problem definition' (1998, p. 32). There may be no point in designing an intervention to improve exercise participation if the local community is already fully engaged in exercise or has other more pressing needs. Information may come from community sources in a variety of ways. As an example with regard to smoking behaviour, a health promotion worker was approached by local health authority workers who were concerned about the number of nursing students taking up smoking. In response, he initiated a survey of nursing students across three training institutions to gather more information about the scope of this problem. Health promoters may initiate needs assessments by other methods which are appropriate to specific questions. These could be the transport needs of older adults, sporting opportunities for young people or a need for support groups for young mothers. Information may be gathered by organizing a survey, focus groups, public meetings or interviews with key informants to ask for information about the community's views on particular health issues; specific groups such as youth, may be surveyed to discover their needs for support to quit smoking or to engage young people in expressing their own perspectives on health issues. Although the name 'community needs assessment' suggests that the origin of the information is the community itself, these activities require some sort of initiating focus. The use of population or local data as evidence for the importance of any health issue is still grounded in particular theories, ideologies and values.

Theoretical approaches to assessing the evidence

It is important to remember that although summaries of findings such as the WHO reports seem clear in print, these data are not cast in stone. Within the disciplines there are always ongoing discussions and disputes about the measurement and meaning of the data reproduced in such reports. Furthermore, as can be seen by the contrast between the *World Health Report* and *The Solid Facts*, the research questions and findings are framed within discourses that construct health in certain ways and position people as certain sorts of subjects (see Petersen and Lupton, 1996). From the subjective perspective, there are multiple discourses on health, and our accounts of health depend on our own location in a historical, social, political and economic context (Eakin et al., 1996). Robertson (1998) gives an example of how epidemiological evidence for the relationship between wealth and health may be used to support different theoretical and ideological approach. One, a 'population health discourse', proposes shifting resources from the health care to the economic sector on the basis of evidence that improving the wealth of a nation improves everybody's health. The other, a 'health promotion discourse', draws on social determinants of health evidence to argue for decreasing inequalities.

The application of understandings from epidemiological data, or the basis of any 'community needs assessment', depends to a large degree on the theoretical and ideological values that health promoters bring to the field. Many of these will be determined by disciplinary practice. Psychology has traditionally promoted itself as a natural science, with a model of research that values 'objective' empirical methods (Bolam and Chamberlain, 2003). In health promotion the focus of this empiricist approach has been on a view of health related behaviours as driven by individual cognitions such as beliefs and attitudes (see Bennett and Murphy, 1997). Thus health psychologists tend to focus on behaviours such as diet, exercise and smoking in terms of the individual cognitions either of particular patients (such as sufferers of COPD or myocardial infarction) or of larger population groups who are to be persuaded to change their attitudes or beliefs and behavioural habits.

Recently, some psychologists have been critical of individual approaches and there have been many suggestions of a shift to an interdisciplinary framework that can include an understanding of the broader social issues in health. For example, Hepworth (2004) suggests that along with the changing nature of public health, and to encompass structural explanations of health, psychologists must shift to a multilevel application of theory and towards interdisciplinary practice. Labonte (2005) describes a multidisciplinary approach to health research which attempts to establish and share theoretical commonalities in a socially oriented approach to health issues. These changing understandings of health promotion across different disciplines lead to reframing of the issues. For example, psychologists who have drawn on Freire's social intervention approach will see psychological and sociopolitical oppression as the central issues rather than particular health related behaviours (Nelson and Prilleltensky, 2005). Prilleltensky and Prillelltensky (2003) have summarized these as moves towards proactive approaches rather than those that are reactive to illness in populations. These authors advocate such proactive approaches to address the underlying social and economic origins of ill health.

The importance of theory and ideology as a basis for these choices will be developed across the following chapters. Preliminary to this development, the next section will consider the broader influences on the choice of issues for health promotion. These myriad influences may be seen as a linked network of different lines bearing down on choices that are made about which determinants of health are the objects of intervention. This network operates like a 'cats cradle' (the game of strings around fingers used to make shapes): shifting the fingers highlights and joins particular lines and makes different shapes. What are the possible lines of influence which foreground particular issues or approaches as important? Those considered here include public health policy, the level of intervention, specific group concerns and the values inherent in all of these.

Public health policy

One very important line of influence on health promotion practice is government health policy. As we noted in Chapter 1, the interest in and influence of governments on public health matters has been the subject of shifting ideologies and discourses. Similar discourses and practices are shared by many countries with similar political, economic and cultural orientations. However, across different countries, a comparison of published public health strategies, shows differences in the development and application of these discourses. An examination of some recent examples of health strategies in countries that are linked by political and historical connection can illustrate these differences. I will describe the examples of Africa, the US, the UK, New Zealand and Sweden in turn.

Countries in Africa

In 2007 the ministers of health of the African Union met in South Africa to develop the 'Africa Health Strategy' (African Union, 2007). The stated goal of this strategy is to contribute to Africa's socioeconomic development by improving the health of its people, especially the poorest and most marginalized, by 2015. The overall objective is to strengthen health systems in order to reduce ill health and accelerate progress towards attainment of this goal. More specifically the aims are:

1 To facilitate the development of initiatives to strengthen national health systems in member states by 2009.
2 To facilitate stronger collaboration between the health and other sectors to improve the socioeconomic and political environment for improving health.
3 To facilitate the scaling up of health interventions in member states including through regional and intergovernmental bodies.

The strategies to achieve these aims include development of health systems (including traditional African health systems), cross-country linkages, addressing poverty and economic development, and evaluation. This document is based on clear understandings of the importance of an infrastructure for the provision of health services and of the barriers to health raised by power imbalances, poverty and the unequal distribution of basic resources such as water and sanitation. At present many health related interventions in Africa continue to focus on individual health behaviours (Barnes, 2007). Many of these interventions are undertaken by non-governmental organizations based in more developed Western countries. Accordingly, the approaches taken reflect the policies, politics and ideologies of those countries.

The United States of America

For example, the US which is one of the most economically developed countries in the world has taken a more disease and illness oriented approach to health issues, which is focused on health behaviours. In January 2000, the US Department of Health and Human Services published *Healthy People 2010* as providing a nationwide health promotion agenda. This strategy, which builds on similar initiatives pursued over the past two decades, is very detailed. It includes 467 objectives designed to serve as guides for improving the health of all people in the United States during the first decade of this century. Each objective has specific targets for improvements to be achieved by the year 2010; for example to reduce cigarette smoking among adults to 12 percent by 2010. The objectives are organized in 28 focus areas, each seen as an important public health area:

1 Access to quality health services.	14 Immunizations and infectious diseases.
2 Arthritis, osteoporosis and chronic back conditions.	15 Injury and violence prevention.
3 Cancer.	16 Maternal, infant and child health.
4 Chronic kidney disease.	17 Medical product safety.
5 Diabetes.	18 Mental health and mental disorders.
6 Disability and secondary conditions.	19 Nutrition and overweight.
7 Educational and community-based programmes.	20 Occupational safety and health.
8 Environmental health.	21 Oral health.
9 Family planning.	22 Physical activity and fitness.
10 Food safety.	23 Public health infrastructure.
11 Health communication.	24 Respiratory diseases.
12 Heart disease and stroke.	25 Sexually transmitted diseases.
13 HIV.	26 Substance abuse.
	27 Tobacco use.
	28 Vision and hearing.

Some of the key objectives have also been included in a limited set known as the 'Leading Health Indicators'. These are: physical activity; overweight and obesity; tobacco use; substance abuse; responsible sexual behaviour; mental health; injury and violence; environmental quality; immunization; and access to health care. This set of objectives is intended to facilitate public comprehension of the importance of health promotion and disease prevention, and to encourage wide participation in improving health. The indicators were chosen based on their effectiveness in motivating action; the availability of data to measure their progress; and their relevance as broad public health issues. I think that this set of key indicators will be familiar as the subject of health promotion messages to most people in Western countries today.

The key objectives are conceived as achievable and measurable changes in the US. The National Centre for Health Statistics (NCHS, see: www.cdc.gov/nchs/about/otheract/hpdata2010/abouthp.htm) is responsible for coordinating the effort to monitor progress towards the objectives, using data from NCHS data systems as well as other sources. National data are gathered from more than 190 different data sources, from federal government departments (health and human services; commerce; education; justice; labour; transportation; and the Environmental Protection Agency), and from voluntary and private non-governmental organizations. Data for some objectives are also provided for subgroups defined by relevant dimensions (such as sociodemographic groups, health status or geographic classifications).

The United Kingdom

The UK has a similar approach to strategies for public health policy but with fewer specific priority areas and a more action oriented approach to the strategy itself. The UK government published a white paper entitled, 'Choosing Health', in 2004 (DoH, 2004) following a four month long consultation period in which some 150,000 people responded directly or took part in local discussions or surveys. The subtitle, 'Making Health Choices Easier', signals a shift towards addressing the practical obstacles to healthy lifestyles, and the white paper identifies six key priorities for health promotion. This strategy has been criticized for being a 'wish list' and not evidence-based. The choice of these overarching priorities is described in the executive summary as being based on both evidence of illness outcomes and public concern about their effects. For example, reducing the number of people who smoke is the first priority because it leads to heart disease, strokes, cancer and many other fatal diseases; because many people felt this was an area in which they needed more support in addressing the problem; because many people were concerned about the affects of secondhand smoke; and because many parents were concerned about their children taking up smoking. The six priority areas are:

1 Reducing the number of people who smoke.
2 Reducing obesity and improving diet and nutrition.
3 Increasing exercise.
4 Encouraging and supporting sensible drinking,
5 Improving sexual health.
6 Improving mental health.

Within each priority area the white paper also outlines a number of legislative, environmental and educational changes aimed at improving public health. For example with regards to reducing obesity the recommendations include action on:

♦ Advertising and promotion of foods to children.
♦ Simplified food labelling and clear labelling to indicate fat, sugar and salt content by mid-2005.
♦ Obesity education and prevention.
♦ Nutritional standards in schools, hospitals and the workplace.
♦ In regard to smoking the paper makes specific promises for government action, for example:
   (i) by the end of 2008 all enclosed public places will be smoke-free: any bar or restaurant preparing and serving food will be smoke-free; and
   (ii) tighter advertising of tobacco and government consultation on using picture warnings on tobacco products.

In all of the priority areas there is also an emphasis on behaviour change and national campaigns, guidelines and information dissemination to encourage changes. This approach has been criticized for renewing the focus on individual lifestyles and reducing the role for government. Hunter (2005) notes that health inequalities receive 'passing mention' and their determinants ignored. In contrast, health is constructed as the sole responsibility of individuals and the importance of community oriented prevention is ignored. Hunter questions whether the problem of widening inequalities in health can be addressed by focusing on individual health behaviours in this way.

New Zealand

Both the US and the UK strategy publications do suggest that the overarching goals of health promotion include eliminating health disparities. However, the objectives themselves are focused on disease and individual behaviours. This narrow focus has been criticized because it does not match the discourse of the objectives. This includes society-wide issues such as unemployment and income inequalities as being important aspects of health. Similarly, in New Zealand, the public health strategy published in 2000 included a rhetorical focus on social inequalities and particularly ethnic inequalities (Ministry of Health, 2000). In New Zealand there is particular concern about health inequalities between Māori who are the original settlers of the country and the now larger and dominant group, descendants of subsequent European settlers. These two groups are partners to a treaty between Māori and the British Crown (representing the second major wave of colonizing settlers). The treaty means that, even if for no other reason, the rights of Māori to participation and equal health must be recognized. More recent updates to the government health strategy include explicit recognition of the effects of colonization, exclusion and racism on Māori health (Ministry of Health, 2002). However, the particular priority issues that have

been noted and which accordingly provide the focus for research and practice remain largely in the areas of disease outcomes and individual
behaviours such as smoking, nutrition, obesity and physical activity. The
ongoing priority areas for Māori gain are seen in relation to behaviours and
diseases such as immunization, hearing, smoking, diabetes, asthma, mental
health, oral health and injury prevention.

In comparison, the Swedish government has made a stronger move
toward addressing the important structural issues that affect inequalities.
These are the sorts of issues that have also been recognized by the members
of the African Union and lead the health ministers to go beyond illness to
emphasize the need for collaboration between the health and *other state
sectors* to improve the social, economic and political environment as a basis
for improved health.

Sweden

In the context of a wealthy country with far fewer specific disease issues, the
Swedes have also taken note of the evidence for inequalities in health as
being based in broader social disparities. The Swedish health policy
(National Institute of Public Health Sweden, 2003) prioritizes the social
structural and population aspects of current evidence for health inequalities.
The overall aim of this policy is to create social conditions that will ensure
good health for the whole population. The national health policy adopted
by the Swedish Ridsdag in 2003 stipulated eleven general objectives:

1 Social and economic security.
2 Influence and participation.
3 Secure and good growing up conditions.
4 A healthy working environment.
5 A good environment and safe products.
6 Health promoting health services.
7 Increased physical activity.
8 Good eating habits and safe food.
9 Reduced tobacco and harmful alcohol consumption; a drug-free
   society.
10 Protection against infectious disease.
11 Safe sexuality.

The policy is similar to others that we have noted so far in that it includes
many of the issues like drugs, tobacco use, sexual and exercise behaviour that
we are familiar with. The differences, reflected in the prioritizing of the first
objectives shows that the aims of the Swedish strategy are based on broader
social and environmental shifts including a reduction of inequalities in
health among groups of different socioeconomic status, gender groups,
ethnic groups and geographical groups. The strategy is accordingly entitled,
'Health on Equal Terms – National Targets for Public Health'.

For the purposes of implementation the strategy is described in terms of 18 national goals for public health. Ohrling (2003) has emphasized that these goals are expressed in terms of *determinants* of health, based on evidence to date rather than as national targets. Through this strategy there is a clear relation between the goals and the political actions required in order to achieve them. One of the effects of the determinants approach is that the focus of public health work is moved beyond the health and medical government sector. If the goals are more broadly accepted by the State (and so by those in housing, transport, welfare and finance policy sectors of government) then they will guide actions in many sectors of the society. To this end, Ohrling also describes how the goals are prioritized in terms of four strategies: integrating health in politics, health oriented community planning, influencing lifestyle and developing public health infrastructure:

Integrating health in politics

1 A strong sense of solidarity and feeling of community in society.
2 A supportive social environment for the individual.
3 Safe and equal conditions in childhood for all children.
4 A high level of employment.
5 A healthy working environment.

Health oriented community planning

6 Accessible green areas for recreation.
7 A healthy in- and outdoor environment.
8 Safe environments and products.

Influencing lifestyle

9 Increased physical activity.
10 Healthy eating habits.
11 Safe sex.
12 Reduced tobacco consumption.
13 Reduced harmful alcohol consumption.
14 A drug-free society.

Public health infrastructure

15 A more health oriented health service.
16 Coordinated public health strategies.
17 Long-term investment in public health methods development, research and training.
18 Access to accurate and objective health information.

A quick comparison of these determinants with the targets of other public health policies will show that although the concern with healthy lifestyles and individual action is retained, there is an additional emphasis on the social and structural aspects of health and well being for all. This shift in the issues of concern to the state may be seen as part of a general move in public health towards concern for underlying social and economic origins of ill health.

Group and local issues

Government policy influences the focus of government bodies, agencies, and researchers and health promoters working for government funded institutions. However, there are many more local or specific concerns to be addressed through a health promotion approach (like tooth brushing, using the rubbish bins, hand washing or prevention of acute respiratory disorders through appropriate medication use). These may well be related to overarching policy but they also arise as issues because of specific needs. For example, many health policies include oral health as an issue, and this issue may take on a particular focus for health workers in a rural area in which many young children have dental caries.

The example of children's teeth also highlights the consideration of particular issues in regard to different sections of the population. If we look at the population by age groups, then different issues are more important for children, adolescents or the elderly. Similarly, other population groups have special issues, such as men or women, and different ethnic or cultural groups. Issues may also be brought to the fore by the active participation of interested or affected groups themselves. For example, self-help groups to support people with particular illnesses have grown into large non-governmental agencies who sponsor research and prevention initiatives. The disability movement for civil rights and autonomy is an example of people working successfully to influence the social, political and physical environment that impacts on the health of people with disabilities. Lines converge from these many different perspectives to point to particular issues for action.

Green et al. (2000, p. 10) suggest that, rather than taking an issues- or population-group-based approach to the 'breadth of roots and expectations' in health promotion, a settings approach is appropriate. This perspective on health promotion is the basis of their book, which covers settings which commonly form a focus for interventions such as: home and family, schools, workplace, health care institutions, clinical settings, community and State. This is a useful way to consider health promotion practice. For example, there are particular issues and practices that are relevant to work place health promotion in regard to both physical and psychological safety. Thus this area alone is the subject of many books and specialized practice. Much health psychology practice also takes place in clinical settings such as hospitals, where the need for prevention of further illness, such as a myocardial infarction, provides a clear site for intervention.

A perspective that could be seen as generating evidence for a focus on issues in particular populations and through particular settings, is the life-course approach (Davey Smith, 2003) to considering inequalities in health. The basis of this approach is an understanding that poor health in later adulthood (such as myocardial infarction) is the result of the combined effects of different material conditions across the lifecourse. Thus a child may experience poor nutrition in utero, a stressful childhood, early pregnancy, poor work conditions and take up smoking, which together impact on later disease outcomes. When lifecourses are understood as a series of potential critical time windows of exposure or as open to the influences of particular life experiences, this approach may be used to determine both the population group vulnerable to and the setting of particular issues. For examples there are particular age groups such as infants, adolescents or the middle aged for which particular aspects of the lifecourse will determine later health outcomes. At the same time, these age groups suggest particular settings such as in schools or doctors' surgeries where the issues are pertinent and the people are accessible.

The shaping of evidence using lifecourse models is based in particular theoretical and ideological explanations of the relationship between deprivation and health that will be described in Chapter 3. At this point I want to simply note that there is always a theoretical basis, and that the issues on which we focus are influenced by that theoretical basis whether we are aware of it or not. An important implication of the theoretical basis of any approach is the level or scope for change chosen for health promotion. Where do we place our concern? Where are the determinants of health located? The shifting emphasis of health promotion from concerns with individual behaviour to broader social concerns often implies different levels at which the issues themselves are understood.

Scope or level for change of the determinants

There are many possible 'levels' at which health issues may be understood. To explain this notion of levels, I will take some examples from an article by Davis et al. (2000) who suggested some directions for public health in New Zealand for the new millennium. These suggestions included different types of public health action: disease prevention, health education, community action and public health policy. I have added the physical environment. Health promotion activities and health psychologists may work with issues specified at any of these levels.

Disease prevention

Health promoters have long contributed to public health work in primary disease prevention. At this level of medical intervention the most obvious example is contributions to the development of vaccination programmes in which the uptake of vaccination for both adults and children is seen as behaviour to be encouraged. Secondary disease prevention is also an important focus at this level. Practices such as screening for diseases and early detection of breast cancer are the kind of issues chosen here.

Health education

Health education has long been an important arena of health promotion activity and an important area for psychologists in particular. At this level the issues are usually those of health behaviour change and influencing people's beliefs about the importance of engaging in particular behaviours like hand washing, eating vegetables or driving safely. These issues may be seen as located in particular groups, settings or populations.

Community action

At this level the specific needs of community members may be foregrounded. However, the issues are also likely to be driven by many other lines of influence such as the concerns of government policy. Thus, the State's requirement to reduce the incidence of diabetes in the population may be addressed in terms of community needs such as provision of support for exercise or of fresh vegetables. The healthy cities project introduced by WHO in 1986 to implement new public health principles at the local level is an example of concerted community action. The WHO Healthy Cities programme engages local governments in health development through a process of political commitment, institutional change, capacity building, partnership-based planning and innovative projects. 'It promotes comprehensive and systematic policy and planning with a special emphasis on health inequalities and urban poverty, the needs of vulnerable groups, participatory governance and the social, economic and environmental determinants of health' (see www.euro.who.int/healthy-cities). The programme provides resources and connections for participants in regard to highlighted environmental, social and behavioural issues including: ageing, air, alcohol drinking, children and young people, city health development planning, community participation, drugs, environmental health, equity and health, health care policy and planning, health impact assessment, housing, mental health, non-communicable diseases, nutrition, physical activity, poverty, sexual health, smoking, social care, socioeconomic determinants of health, sustainable development, transport and health, urban governance, urban planning, and violence. The issues themselves are little different from others we have reviewed. However, the emphasis on participation, on capacity development of the participating citizens, and the social determinants of health is relatively new.

The environment

The Healthy Cities movement programme includes a concern with the urban environment and the impact of living conditions on health. Health promoters are increasingly recognizing the impact of the physical environment on health behaviours. For example, there is little point in teaching young people to use condoms if condoms are not available nearby. The messages about healthy eating are obviated by the availability and prominence of fatty and sugary food and the serving of larger portions of food. Exhortations to exercise are obviated in an area with no pavements, no parks and dangerous walk ways. To include these broader changes many health promoters have been encouraged to move outside their own disciplinary areas. To work towards the provision of healthy public spaces and healthy housing they must work alongside local government and housing authorities. This move in turn leads to greater concern with the influence of public policy on all these matters. One of the major public health triumphs of the last few decades has been a significant reduction in cigarette smoking. However, this reduction has not been the result of health education messages and health promotion persuasion alone. A large part of the impact on population behaviour has resulted from environmental changes in the availability of cigarettes and cigarette advertising, the cost of cigarettes through taxation, and legislation providing for smoke-free eating and drinking places in many countries. It has become apparent that in the case of this particular behaviour, government policy and legislation has been effective.

The social environment

A large part of the move away from cigarette smoking by many people has also been a move in publicly expressed attitudes to smoking as a damaging behaviour and a corresponding shift in the political will for change. Health related behaviours are influenced by dominant socially shared discourses that give meaning to health behaviours and the nature of health and illness (Petersen and Lupton, 1996). Many of these discourses such as those drawn upon to construct mentally ill people as dangerous, overweight people as morally deficient or illness as being an individual's fault, are shared and developed through the media (Lyons, 2000). This broader social arena is an important area for action in which issues like understandings of mental illness sufferers or the constructions of particular racial groups may be seen to have serious effects on health.

Public policy

Davis et al. (2000) suggested that, given the recent shifts in the focus of health promotion, understanding the issues at public policy level is very important. 'Yet, such higher level policy activities require substantial political commitment and social support' (2000, p. 3). Nevertheless, it is becoming apparent that this is an important level of effective action for health promoters. The potential for influence is through published health strategies that direct all publicly funded workers, the provision of state funding to important areas of practice, the potential of legislation and economic distribution for reducing inequities, and the importance of other areas of state influence (e.g., housing, recreational areas, transport, employment and social welfare) to health. The issues that may be most usefully affected through government policy are the broader social and economic issues such as income inequality, stress in early life, unemployment and exclusion, that evidence currently suggests are having the most reliable and damaging effects on health. Wilkinson and Marmot (2006), present a summary of this evidence to highlight the importance of the role that public policy can play in shaping a social environment that is more conducive to better health. These issues can also be considered in terms of international policy. As Marks (2004) has noted, poverty, powerlessness and inequality are international health issues.

Although it may be useful to consider the different levels of focus for descriptive purposes, Crossley (2002) has pointed out that a focus on health related issues in isolation is problematic. She describes that ways in which health promotion practice focuses on individual health behaviour issues such as smoking, poor diet, poor health care and risky sexual practices, without taking into account the relationships between these behaviours, which would necessarily lead to consideration of broader social factors. Labonte (2005) also points to the limitations of understanding categories of health determinants as separate. In describing a model of public health that includes levels of health determining conditions, he says that understanding the relationships between such levels is as important as considering the issues themselves.

The level or levels at which health issues are defined in practice has implications for strategies, outcomes, social policies and priorities. In practice we cannot work at all levels, so how do we decide what are the important ways to choose? Seedhouse (1997) describes how in practice these choices often happen in an ad hoc, undertheorized and conflicting manner. He also suggests that the values of health promoters are the basis of choices of focus. When health researchers, theorists and practitioners in the field address their personal, disciplinary and political values, the ways in which all such decisions are value driven becomes more apparent.

The values of health promotion

Health promoters are often oblivious of the cultural values that are embedded in the choice of issues for health promotion. At every point of the process, from evidence to practice, choices are made that reflect the dominant values of the researchers and practitioners and the prevailing ideology of their society. The importance of values means that at each step in the process of developing health promotion activities there are ethical issues to be considered. This consideration should begin with the choice of and approach to the health issues of concern. Why do we want people to quit smoking? Is it for their personal well being, our well being (in terms of physical health, distaste or moral beliefs about addiction), or is the basic concern to relieve the burden on the health care system and the tax payer? 'Even advice about diet and exercise is never based wholly on fact. At some stage a value judgement of some kind will be made' (Seedhouse, 1998, p. xiii). Seedhouse (1997) goes further to say that there are two contradictory tenets of health promotion practice: (1) that evidence drives health promotion; or (2) that values drive health promotion. The first view is held by government and other official health promoters, the news media, the general public, many health promotion practitioners and health promotion theorists. Seedhouse suggests that some of these groups will accept that values are involved, and theorists usually want to include the values-driven understanding as well. However, he argues that health promotion cannot be driven by both values and evidence: it is driven primarily by values. According to this perspective, the particular values and political philosophies of health promoters are the very first step in paying attention to any health issue. From this position decisions about what is an issue for concern and the evidence for its existence are chosen.

Following these sorts of understandings about the central importance of values, Guttman (2000) suggests a values-based evaluation of all health promotion activities rather than a strategic basis. She has critically analysed the values involved in several facets of health promotion which also involve ethical considerations. She notes that these values and ethical issues may be invisible if we take it for granted that the purpose of health promotion activities is only to do good. An uncritical assumption that health promotion activities are an unalloyed virtue means that possible harmful effects are not considered. Apparently desirable objectives such as changing risky behaviours should be open to ongoing questioning and examination. For example, Crossley (2002) has explored the suggestion that some contemporary health messages are actually promoting risky health practices through people's resistance to restrictions on their autonomy. In responding to what seems like relentless attempts to control their behaviour (in the very complex moral environment of AIDS and gay sex) some men are actively resisting messages promoting condom use and other aspects of 'safe sex'. There are now several other examples of health promotion activities that have created harm in some way and Guttman (2000) provides a very structured analytic approach to bringing the values implicit in any intervention planning to the fore and considering the ethical issues they may raise. Those areas raised by Guttman that are relevant to choosing a health issue for change include the way a health related issue is defined; the particular way an issue is framed; the understandings of causes of health related problems; and the values of the health promoters themselves. The values involved in these different facets will necessarily underpin the goals of an intervention. I will consider some examples of each in turn.

Defining the health issue

A health issue is defined as a problem by certain groups or organizations. When governments decide on the focus for public health strategies, they are influenced by their own ideologies and the influence of powerful lobby groups and other interests. The way an issue is defined reflects the values and priorities of those who describe it. Values shape the ways in which problems are perceived and who is perceived as a problem.

The important issue of health inequalities is an overt example of these differences. There is powerful and persuasive epidemiological evidence that shows differences in health and mortality related to social and economic position. Nevertheless, the explanations for this evidence are controversial. In particular, two groups of public health researchers currently provide competing broad approaches to explanations. The 'neo-materialists' argue for the importance of housing, environment and material conditions of life across the lifespan. Others have focused on psychosocial explanations (such as exclusion, control and stress) for the differences. Both approaches have implications for public health policy and interventions (see Chapter 3). Although the arguments between these two groups bring the ideological basis of the neo-materialist claims into the debate, the assumptions behind many other issues are not so often challenged. Whaley (2003) says that '. . . epidemiologists, like most human beings, may not necessarily be aware of the influences of the dominant cultural ideology on the way they conduct and interpret their research'. The importance of culture as an all-encompassing context for human behaviour and the values that influence practice is 'likely either to be ignored or taken for granted' (2003, p. 740).

Guttman raises the example of adolescent pregnancy, which is currently seen in most medical, social policy, and popular literature as a problem. Today, if we read a mainstream newspaper headline featuring 'teenage pregnancy' or 'adolescent mothers' we do not need any gloss to know that the headline is flagging a 'problem'. However, the age at which women have children has been a matter of changing historical and cultural definition, and is currently subject to a range of moral, social and economic values. Particular concerns and definitions of 'the problem' will differ depending on moral stances regarding premarital sex. It will also depend on whether health promoters see the issue in regard to health outcomes for the children; or in regard to the well being of adolescent parents (who may be seen as suffering interrupted development from one cultural perspective); or as an economic demand on a society which must support the young mothers. These differing definitions of the issue of adolescent motherhood will have an impact on the way that people see young mothers, on young mothers' perceptions of themselves and on their relationship with health care providers (Breheny and Stephens, 2007).

Whaley (2003) also points out the importance of the level at which an issue is defined. Individual level approaches in epidemiology have value laden and political implications because such analyses have seen broader issues at the social or political level as outside consideration for intervention. Thus, important cultural understandings of the basis of certain health issues are ignored in the dominant approach which emphasizes individual level variation.

Framing the health issue

Public health messages may be based on certain ideologies or models of causation that are not examined in relation to other explanations. There may be implicit claims or distorted representations in the ways that the health issue is translated into health promotion messages. Guttman uses the example of heart disease which has been presented to the public in many Western countries as preventable through individual lifestyle changes such as exercise and diet. The definition of the problem includes assumptions that people will exercise if motivated, and ignores other known factors in heart disease such as differences in working conditions. Messages based on these assumptions also include the implicit message that exercise, diet and cardiovascular health predict heart disease, and that there are no other or unknown factors in its aetiology (although these factors predict only a small proportion of the risk according to epidemiological evidence).

Similarly, the evidence for the efficacy of preventive screening such as mammograms is often simplified, for the well meaning purpose of reducing confusion (e.g., Kahl and Lawrence-Bauer, 1996). These health promoters actively oppose the publication of any knowledge that may present alternative views. They believe this will confuse the clarity of the issue they want presented in a particular way.

However, such distorted representations may be unethical because they deny the public certain knowledge, and bias the messages in the direction desired by the educators. The difficulties arising from this approach are two layered. First, the health promoters have not examined their own assumptions about the value of such deception and have not faced the basic ethical dilemma in this choice. Second, the ethical dilemma is simply not recognized because the health promoters have taken on this approach to framing the health issue without critical consideration; they believe that they have chosen the best approach on behalf of other women.

The use of research that is framed in a particular way will provide evidence that serves to perpetuate dominant cultural stereotypes and social injustice. Whaley (2003) describes how the use of epidemiological evidence of health disparities to classify individuals as being at risk on the basis of their ethnicity or race raises ethical concerns. Such classifications are recursive. They are based on unexamined assumptions about the basis of race or ethnicity and serve to stigmatize certain groups. This stigmatization feeds back into the sociocultural processes of rascist societies that maintain social disadvantage. For example, racist discourses that construct Māori people in New Zealand as uniformly pursuing certain health related behaviours have been shown to be drawn upon by well meaning physicians to explain health inequalities (McCreanor and Nairn, 2002).

Understandings of the causes of health issues

There are different ways of understanding the causes of health related problems and different approaches to explanation reflect different sets of values. Guttman shows how explanations at different levels of analysis can reveal the values inherent in the explanation. For example, at the individual level, the suggestion that junk food advertisements on television may affect children's diet seems neutral. The values implicit in this suggestion are hidden because the social structure and market ideologies behind the explanation are taken for granted. At another level, suggesting that junk food ads on television should be banned 'sounds value-laden and political' (Guttman, 2000, p.18) because it questions current structural arrangements and the rights of commercial entities.

There are many similar examples in which a shift from the individual level of explanation (people need to be motivated to exercise) to a physical or social environmental level (people need places to exercise and people need time to exercise) will reveal the values inherent in the explanation (people are lazy or people are constrained). Considering the possibilities of alternative or additional explanations for the causes of a health issue is an important beginning to understanding the assumptions behind the possible explanations and any ethical issues raised by the choice of particular explanations.

The values of the health promoters

The cultural and ideological basis of a health issue that is considered as the basis for intervention should be understood and brought into open and explicit consideration. Guttman (2000) suggests that it is common for health promoters to study the values of the population who will be the target of persuasion or other attempts to influence their attitudes and change their behaviour. However, the values that underly any intervention itself are not usually studied. She gives the example of providing information on food labels as a strategy focus in a cholesterol education programme. The choice of this strategy and the neglect of others, such as changes in the marketplace or workplace, reflect the biomedical orientation of the institution running the programme.

In other situations, differing values (e.g., between health promoters and the community) may cause overt tensions or anomalies. For example, schools may adopt sexual health education programmes in which students are taught how to use condoms. However, the school stakeholders will not condone any additional interventions, such as the provision of free condoms or the placement of condom vending machines in the school (which could make the lessons useful according to the educators), because such apparent encouragement of sexual activity contradicts prevailing values. There is a similar tension around the provision of free and accessible needle exchange facilities for intravenous drug users. These programmes have been demonstrated to help prevent the spread of HIV/AIDS through needle sharing. However, some communities are not prepared to accept any encouragement of illegal and immoral practices that these facilities seem to provide. In these sorts of situations any conflict of values, such as between health workers who advocate needle sharing and the community, raise ethical dilemmas. Whose values and rights should have precedence in these situations?

The goals of the intervention

The choice of a health related issue for which some change is warranted, the definition and framing of the issue, the understandings of its causes and the values of the health promoters and other stake holders will contribute towards the goals of an intervention. What is to be the target for change? And from a values analysis perspective, what values are reflected in these goals? Who does the choice of particular goals for change serve? HIV/AIDS is a worldwide health problem, and across many different countries the goals chosen for AIDS education programmes reflect the dominant values of the state and religious leaders. Guttman (2000) provides examples of many different parts of the world in which the provision of explicit information about practices that could prevent the transmission of infection runs counter to local cultural and religious mores that prohibit sexually explicit information, particularly information related to homosexual or extramarital sexual relations and intravenous drug use or the use of condoms. Hence many messages have focused on the prohibition of or abstinence from these practices and failed to provide explicit information about how to avoid transmission. An additional effect of these campaigns was the stigmatization of certain groups (such as gay men) as the carriers of disease, and a neglect of the risk to women (Welch et al., 1996).

The values of the health promoters can result in quite different goals for intervention. Take two hypothetical models for a programme that is designed to promote the vaccination of children. In one, a biomedical model means that vaccination of all children is valued as the paramount goal. This goal usually leads to a campaign in which parents are taught (in some way) about the merits of vaccination. Alternatively, if the values are community-based then the goal may be empowerment of community members. This goal is more likely to lead to a programme in which parents are taught about their responsibility for their children's health outcomes and how to make decisions about issues like vaccination. An example of the role of unexamined values in choosing goals comes from a discussion among health promotion students about the issue of dog bites. The discussion was based on evidence from council workers in the area of concern to whom dog bites were a growing issue. According to these reports, the dog bites were underreported and undertreated because the dog owners did not want to draw attention to their dangerous dogs. In addition, the local council members were suppressing the evidence because it would make the area undesireable for more affluent house buyers and property developers. The initial suggestions from the student health workers involved a focus on educating the local dog owners about dog care and training. In considering the pragmatics of this approach, they included the understanding that the people were living in largely low income housing. This led to a group member raising questions about the socioeconomic status of the people in the area and the meaning of dog ownership to these people. Once the students began to examine the values involved they were able to question the goal of education based on middle class values of dog control, and to consider new questions about the structural and experiential nature of people's lives; the role of the city council in this problem; and alternative goals.

Ethical issues

A values-based approach foregrounds the moral and political basis of health promotion choices, but does not necessarily mean that we must accept all values as equal. 'It is necessary to hold at least some values to promote anything' and the way forward is to admit the political and moral basis of practice and make choices about values (Seedhouse, 1997, p. 81). When the underlying values in the selection of health issues are highlighted and considered then ethical dilemmas may arise. We have already noted the dilemma of conflicting values when needle exchange programmes or interventions that apparently permit teenagers to engage in sex are suggested. There are a range of such conflicts related to the choice of issues alone.

In considering the solution of ethical dilemmas the principles of bioethics – beneficence (doing good); non-malfeasance (not doing harm); autonomy (people's right to choose); and justice (fair and equitable treatment for all) – may be used to guide us in the first instance. These four principles are commonly applied as the criteria for judgement of the ethical aspects of any health related practice. For example, in regard to justice, questions arise regarding who gets targeted or who the choice of issue will benefit. Information about health practices and preventing disease have been shown to be more accessible by those of higher socioeconomic status. There is also consistent evidence that in many parts of the world public subsidies for health or education intended to promote equity are largely captured by the middle class (Feachem, 2000). Health behaviour recommendations including refraining from smoking, exercising, and eating fruit and vegetables have been more easily taken up by the middle classes, who have the resources to follow the advice. Thus, in several ways, interventions to promote individual health behaviour can benefit those who are already better off and so increase inequalities. A further ethical issue that arises is malefeasance. Health promoters must consider what harms may arise from the choice of issue and the way it is framed. By targeting certain groups as examples of bad health practice any subsequent campaign or policy may serve to stigmatize those groups. For example gay men have been additionally stigmatized by early HIV/AIDS public health communications. Television advertisements showing the results of careless driving may also stigmatize wheelchair users. Public policies targeting people with poorer health can stigmatize certain ethnic groups. An early and systematic examination of the values behind such choices will help to reveal ethical problems.

Reflexivity

The application of ethical principles may be only so much lip service if it is not accompanied by a serious consideration of our own and others' values. We have already noted that it is easy for health promoters to believe that health promotion, in other words, work for the benefit of improved health for others, is a 'good' in its own right if they do not critically consider the basis of this belief. Furthermore, Hisamichi (2004) points out that although the principles of beneficence, non-malfeasance, autonomy and justice appear to reflect universal values, ethics may differ depending on 'religion, race, region, national history, level of scientific technology, and the economic situation . . . Something that is considered "good" in Japan may be considered "not good" in another country, or vice versa' (p. 110). Or, as Whaley (2003) has said, 'ethics converge with culture on the notion of values' and their influence on practice. The choices made in the face of ethical dilemmas reflect both the ethical and cultural background that underlies the value system of a practitioner (p. 740). Accordingly, the principle of reflexivity comes into play. That is, practitioners need to be able to understand their own cultural standpoint, recognize that there are values inherent in their moral and political position; that these will influence their understandings of health related practice; and be prepared to recognize where these values differ from those of other groups. Bolam and

Chamberlain (2003) maintain that reflexivity should be central to critical health psychology practice. They add that reflexivity should include ongoing questioning of the political, moral, ethical and sociohistorical context of practice. Such questioning has the potential for infinite regression and paralysis. Chamberlain (2004) addresses this issue and suggests that reflexivity should seen as a recognition that values, assumptions, ethics and practice are all bound up together and 'reflexivity provides a means to determine a coherent stance in relation to them' (p. 134). To express the practical importance of such a stance, Labonte et al. (2005), in writing about population health research, have lucidly summarized the key elements of a values-based approach to any health related practice:

> A critical approach to population health research is as unavoidably moral as it is inherently political. Its praxis – a reflective cycle of action informed by theory/evidence/values – challenges its practitioners to blur the boundaries between their personal and the work/career lives. Morality without evidence risks righteousness; evidence without a moral base risks passivity.

Summary

This chapter has focused on the question of what makes some aspects of health an issue for concern and how certain determinants of health become the focus of intervention. It turns out that from different perspectives there are myriad influences on these choices. I have outlined different sources of evidence for health concerns and their determinants, and how different theoretical approaches influence the interpretation and application of that evidence. Research evidence both contributes to and interacts with other lines of influence that may combine in different ways to highlight particular health issues. I have pointed to the influence of government policy, particular group concerns and the different levels of intervention at which the issue is conceptualized. Interwoven through these lines of influence are the values of stakeholders, researchers and health promoters. Values are always the basis of choice but often unexamined.

Seedhouse (1997) has suggested that the values of health promoters are the driving force behind practice including the interpretation of evidence and use of theory. Labonte et al. (2005) have described a moral and political praxis involving theory, evidence and values in a reflexive cycle, in which each is recursively essential to the other. Whichever way we attempt to explain these processes we realize the difficulties and artificiality of separating out different aspects for consideration on their own. Nevertheless, since it is difficult to capture this interrelatedness, in the following chapters I will focus on evidence, theory and methods in turn, while asking you to bring your own values and position to a critical evaluation of the material at each step.

In Chapter 3, I will consider the evidence for unequal health outcomes across populations, and then in subsequent chapters, some of the theoretical and methodological bases available for understanding these and other observations, and for developing a focus for interventions. Along the way we will consider the values implied by certain choices and the ethical implications of those choices at each step of practice in health promotion.

Further reading

1 In this chapter I have drawn heavily from the books of particular authors whose work I recommend be read in their own right:

Guttman, N. (2000) *Public Health Communication Interventions: Values and Ethical Dilemmas*. Thousand Oaks, CA: Sage.

Petersen, A. and Lupton, D. (1996) *The New Public Health: Health and Self in the Age of Risk*. London: Sage.

Seedhouse, D. (1997) *Health Promotion: Philosophy, Prejudice and Practice*. Chichester: John Wiley & Sons.

Seedhouse, D. (1998) *Ethics: The Heart of Health Care*, 2nd edn. Chichester: John Wiley & Sons.

2 For more information on different approaches to needs assessment which has been covered briefly in this chapter:

Annett, H. and Rifkin, S.B. (1995) *Guidelines for Rapid Participatory Appraisals to Assess Community Health Needs: A Focus on Health Improvements for Low Income Urban and Rural Areas*. Geneva: World Health Organization.

Misra, R. and Ballard, D. (2003) Community needs and strengths assessment as an active learning project, *The Journal of School Health*, 73, 269–71.

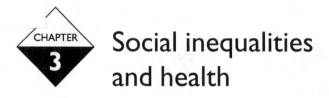

Social inequalities and health

Introduction

Social inequalities are reflected across all the major health issues of developed countries today. Evidence shows that differences in income, education, social class or ethnicity are related to inequalities in illnesses, health care, health related behaviours and mortality. The powerful evidence showing that poverty is still related to poor health in poor and wealthy countries is concerning but not surprising. The remarkable aspect of the socioeconomic status (SES) and health relationship is that there are differences across all levels of any hierarchy of income or status so that even inequalities between very wealthy people have been shown to be related to differences in health. Social groupings that reflect social status, especially ethnicity, are an important aspect of these inequalities. In regard to health promotion interventions there is a need to understand the basis of this observed relationship between social inequalities and health. However, the reasons are still not well understood, despite decades of research attention. In this chapter, I will outline the basis of the evidence and the controversies about its interpretation.

The choice of inequalities as the example of a health issue in this chapter has been influenced by the values of a critical approach to health psychology. Prilleltensky and Prillelltensky (2003) suggest that focusing attention at the level of individual wellness alone, without considering broader social issues, is ineffective. A social perspective that includes understandings of the impact of disadvantage and oppression is important in developing critical knowledge of the roles of power and inequality in health. From this broader social perspective, inequalities in health have become a central issue for policymakers and health promoters. Inequalities in health outcomes across social groups lead health promoters to consider the interaction of the material, psychological, social, moral and political aspects of physical and mental health.

Poverty and health

Poverty or material deprivation is well understood as the major cause of ill health. Decreases in poverty in developed countries have been widely shown to be more important to health than any improvements in medical care, and poverty is accepted as the most important social determinant of health (Nguyen and Peschard, 2003). The demonstrated mechanisms by which poverty is understood to cause disease are easy to understand. The material deprivation of absolute poverty causes weakened immunity and neurophysiological development through malnutrition, the spread of diseases is enhanced by poor living conditions, and increased environmental pollutants also threaten well being. These are problems that many governments, non-governmental agencies (NGOs), and the World Health Organization (WHO) grapple with today in many poor countries of the world.

Social inequalities and health

The epidemiological transition

In more developed countries the population has shifted through what Richard Wilkinson (2005) describes as the 'epidemiological transition'. This refers to a move from large numbers of people living in absolute material poverty to a situation in which basic needs are met for the whole population. Within these populations there are still groups living in conditions of relative poverty. The epidemiological shift is reflected in marked changes in population health status. For example, further increases in wealth across the whole population are no longer reflected in improvements in health. In the richest countries of the world there is little relation between increases in living standards (even twofold) and population life expectancy. Additionally, in populations which have moved through this shift, the importance of infectious diseases as causes of illness and death declines to be replaced by chronic illnesses and degenerative diseases as the chief concerns. Conditions that were once a problem for wealthy people, like coronary health disease (CHD), obesity, and even gout, become the diseases of the poorer groups in society. Wilkinson suggests that for public health researchers, this shift from grappling with problems of meeting basic physical needs in developed countries has revealed the importance of the psychosocial aspects of health, in addition to the effects of material deprivation.

Social status is related to health

One of the important signals that drew public health research attention to these aspects was *The Black Report and the Health Divide* (Townsend et al., 1986) which drew on evidence from Europe and the US, to point to growing inequalities in health related directly to inequalities in social class. One of the key studies contributing to this evidence is the longitudinal Whitehall study (Marmot et al., 1984), which showed that inequalities in age of mortality, among a group of 18,403 men employed in the British civil service, were related to a social hierarchy, measured as occupational grades. Men from the lowest grade of occupation died earlier on average than those from the highest grade. Moreover, and this is the most important aspect of these findings, the life expectancy of the men increased with each step higher in the hierarchy (from support staff, through clerical and professional executive, to administrative). This gradient, in which the mortality risk decreases with each small step up the social ladder, is best understood as a graph (see Figure 3.1). The Whitehall study was originally intended to study coronary heart disease (CHD), not social inequalities at all; occupational grade was the only social indicator in the study, and the findings were unexpected. Nevertheless, the findings were the same for mortality from CHD, cancers, cardiovascular and respiratory diseases, gastrointestinal diseases, violence, accidents and suicide.

Evidence for the gradient is robust

Most public health researchers now take this relationship as a given. The recognition that social inequalities are directly related to health inequalities are accepted as robust because they have been observed in many different

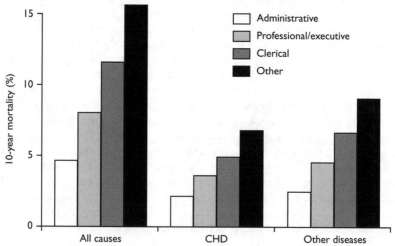

Figure 3.1 Age adjusted mortality rates by grade of employment for civil servants aged 40–64 in the Whitehall Study (%)

Source: From Marmot and Davey Smith, 1997; reproduced by permission of Sage Publications Ltd.

situations, across different sorts of health outcomes, and using different measures to tap social status. First, similar results have been found in populations in wealthy countries: the UK, the US, Canada, Finland, Japan, France, Sweden, Germany, Italy, Belgium, Australia and New Zealand (Marmot, 2004). They have also been found within other social groupings such as in women (Marmot et al., 1991) or within different ethnic groups (Tobias and Yeh, 2006). Second, gradients show up when either mortality or morbidity in the main causes of death and disease is measured (Townsend et al., 1986; Marmot, 2004). Third, the Whitehall findings have been reproduced whether researchers use income, material assets, education, parent's social class or area level deprivation as proxies for social position (Carroll and Davey Smith, 1997; Marmot, 2004).

Social status affects everybody

The observations of British civil servants provide compelling evidence, but there are other engaging observations that reinforce our understandings of the historical nature of the gradient. That is, the gradient has long existed even when not so well recognized. They also hammer home the point that the differences in health and life expectations are found between fine grained levels of social status, and between groups of wealthy people, not just among deprived groups.

Carroll et al. (1996) describe two historical studies. In the city of Florence in the fifteenth century, affluent fathers could deposit dowry investments against their daughters' marriage. The city also kept records of citizen deaths. Comparisons of the size of a woman's dowry with her age at death show a gradient of increasing age of mortality from the larger dowries down to the smaller.

A second even more inventive example from these authors describes a study of the height of commemorative obelisks in a Glaswegian cemetery in the nineteenth century. This study was based on the assumption that the taller the obelisk, the wealthier the family of the deceased. Again, these were all relatively affluent people, who had lived longer than the average for their day and whose occupations were largely professional. Nevertheless, comparisons revealed a clear gradient in the relationship between height and age of death: the taller the obelisk, the longer the life.

Marmot also provides examples of the gradient's operation among wealthy people today. Sweden is an egalitarian country and this is reflected in a shallower gradient than in other countries. Nevertheless, research has shown that across a hierarchy of educational qualifications, those with PhDs live longer than those with Master's degrees, who live longer than those with Bachelor degrees, and so on as the qualification levels decrease (Wilkinson and Marmot, 2006).

Equally intriguing and more dramatic is the report of a US study of film actors who had all been nominated for motion picture Academy Awards.

The researchers compared the winners with the losers, reasoning that apart from this difference in social status, there was no difference in wealth. The Oscar winners lived a remarkable four years longer than their co-stars who were nominated but did not win! Marmot (2004) points to the import of this difference by calculating that if there was no coronary heart disease, the average population life expectancy would increase by just under four years.

Inequalities between societies

Once researchers began to take more notice of social inequalities, it became evident that the health and wealth differences themselves vary between different societies and across history (Wilkinson, 2005). Some societies are more unequal than others. The first implication of these comparisons is to reinforce understandings that the effects on health are caused by people's relative social position, not just by absolute deprivation. Thus, people in a wealthy society with access to clean running water, refrigerators, televisions and sufficient food may be much better off physically than people in earlier times or in a poorer country. But because they are relatively poor in their own society, their health is worse (Nguyen and Peschard, 2003).

A second implication concerns differences in the steepness of the gradient. Many public health researchers are concerned about growing inequalities between the top and bottom of the gradient. For example, in England and Wales, the differences between the mortality rates in relation to social class for men have increased steadily between 1950 and the 1990s (Carroll and Davey Smith, 1997), in other words, the gradient for these countries is becoming steeper. Similarly, growing inequalities have been observed in the US, New Zealand, Finland and other Western industrialized countries with a related widening of socioeconomic status differences in health (MacIntyre and Hunt, 1997; Williams et al., 1997).

Epidemiologists making comparisons across countries have pointed to an additional finding in regard to these differences in the gaps between the poor and the rich, and the related health inequalities. The greater the social or economic inequalities, the worse the health of the *whole* population. Wilkinson (2005) has reproduced data to support the suggestion that the size of the gaps in relative income and social status within countries is related to health inequalities between countries. For example, the US is one of the wealthiest countries and spends far more per person on health care than any other country. At the same time it is the most unequal in income differences of the developed countries and is only twenty-fifth on international rankings of life expectancy. Similarly, Britain's growing income inequalities are related to a drop in life expectancy ranking. Wilkinson also draws on studies across cities in the world to show that cities in the more equitable countries of Sweden and Australia have lower mortality rates than cities in the US and Britain. Countries with medium sized economies such as South Africa and Brazil have vast inequalities in social and economic indicators along with very poor health statistics (Sanders and Chopra, 2006). These findings are not always as clear as suggested in this brief account and there are anomalies and critiques of this line of research (Lynch et al., 2003; Wilkinson and Pickett, 2006). However, the implications of a growing body of evidence from this line of enquiry is that at the same absolute level of material wealth, people in a more egalitarian country will be healthier than one in a less egalitarian society (Nguyen and Peschard, 2003). These growing social inequalities are seen as unjustly resulting in worse health for those at the bottom of the social gradient, as causing preventable illness and death, and as a situation that is clearly open to change.

Racial and ethnic inequalities

Deaton and Lubotsky (2003) have critiqued findings relating to inequalities between US states, claiming that observed health differences are related to race, not income. Exworthy et al. (2006) have suggested that the focus on differences, whether on economic differences or racial differences, is in relation to the concerns of the particular society. In countries like the US it is racial inequalities that are the most apparent problem, whereas in other countries class or area inequalities come to the fore. The US has several minority ethnic groups who have poorer health in general than the white population, including Native Americans (the indigenous people from several nations), Asians, Pacific Islanders, African Americans and Hispanics. There are well documented inequalities between these racial or ethnic minority groups, particularly between the largest group of African Americans and the white majority. African Americans have had higher rates of death, disease and disability for over 150 years (Williams et al., 1997). Byrd and Clayton (2003) note that currently, 'African Americans are faced with persistent or worsening, wide and deep, race-based health disparities compared with either the white or the general population' (p. 477). These inequalities are usually found across all measures of socioeconomic status, such as education, occupation and income, as well as all aspects of health. Accordingly questions are raised about the interaction of these factors, about which is a proxy for which in large scale studies, and whether for example, socioeconomic status or income is a pathway, or control variable, or of no account (e.g., Williams et al., 1997; Lynch et al., 2003).

Whatever the theoretical perspective, most findings show that in considering individual level data (not countries or states) a large part of the ethnicity and health relationship may be explained by income or other measures of socioeconomic status. However, there remains an additional effect of race or ethnicity on health that cannot be explained by the other measures of social status. Many commentators consider that the additional underlying factor is racism, whether structural, institutional or interpersonal. To explore this suggestion, Williams et al. (1997) compared self-reports of stress and experiences of unfair discrimination reported by 520 white and 586 black respondents in a US survey of health and socioeconomic status. As expected, the racial differences in health were reduced when adjusted for education and income. Additionally, perceived discrimination and stress explained further differences in health status. The measures of discrimination were self-report and probably captured a very limited picture of the sorts of daily experiences of discrimination that people (both black and white) actually notice, without addressing the broader, taken for granted and subtle forms of racism in society (McCreanor and Nairn, 2002; Geiger, 2003; Good et al., 2003). Given these limitations, the results provide support for the direct role of discrimination on health.

New Zealand is another country in which racial inequalities are an important issue and a matter for government concern and intervention. New Zealand's indigenous population, the Māori, have been in the minority since colonization by British settlers in the late nineteenth century. On average, Māori also show marked differences in all areas of health when compared to the majority group, who are of European extraction. Across the whole population the familiar gradient may be observed: the unequal distribution of income, education, employment and housing is directly related to health inequalities (Woodward et al., 2000). Tobias and Yeh (2006) examined the four main ethnic groups in New Zealand separately and showed that there are deprivation gradients on all-cause mortality for Asian, Pacific Island, Māori and European. However, the gradients for these groups have different slopes with Māori having twice the mortality rate of non–Māori and non–Pacific people, and Pacific people (mostly migrants from the Pacific Islands) in between the two (Blakely et al., 2006). In considering differences among Māori, Sporle et al. (2002) have shown that the social class mortality gradient is much stronger for Māori than for non–Māori (see Figure 3.2). Māori are represented across each social class (measured by occupation), but within each social class mortality is markedly higher for Māori. An agreement in this literature at present is that inequalities in income, education and housing (Blakely et al., 2005) are the primary cause of health inequalities. However, there are additional factors that contribute to ethnic health inequalities (e.g., Ministry of Health, 2002; Sporle, 2002; Blakely et al., 2006). Suggested additional reasons for these disparities include the effects of colonization and land confiscation, structural and interpersonal racism, unequal access to good quality health services and differences in risky health behaviours such as smoking (Ministry of Health, 2002; Blakely et al., 2006). Harris et al. (2006) used survey questions about verbal attacks, physical attacks and unfair treatment by a health professional, at work, or when buying or renting housing to demonstrate the experience of racial discrimination and deprivation on health outcomes in New Zealand. Māori were more likely to report discrimination in all instances and were almost ten times more likely to experience discrimination in three or more settings than Europeans. These experiences explained some of the variance

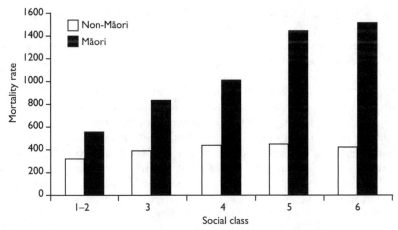

Figure 3.2 New Zealand male age standarized mortality rates (per 100,000 person years) by occupationally defined social class and ethnicity, 1996–97

Source: From Sporle, Pearce and Davis, 2002; reproduced with permission from *The New Zealand Medical Journal.*

in various health outcomes, leading the researchers to conclude that racism, both interpersonal and institutional, contributes to inequalities in health between Māori and Europeans in New Zealand.

A focus on the health inequities for people marked by colour or ethnicity, who have histories of racial and ethnic discrimination, injustice, colonization and exclusion, highlights the importance of this social factor. In many ways ethnic differences are closely aligned with all the other differences in income, education and social class that have been observed in many societies. The suggested effects of racism and discrimination may be seen as stronger or more blatant expressions of the hierarchical structure of many societies today. These most clearly discriminatory rankings provide us with the greatest concern about injustices in health outcomes, and also more evidence for the effects of psychosocial factors on health. Qualitative investigations into these social factors from anthropology and social psychology suggest that clear markers such as ethnicity define the responses of those in power and act as a marker for social status and differences between dominant and repressed groups in society. For example, in the health care field alone, both Good et al. (2003) in the US and McCreanor and Nairn (2002) in New Zealand have shown how even well meaning health care professionals unintentionally reproduce racist categorizations and marginalizing experiences of ethnic minority groups.

There is an additional point to consider about ethnicity across different countries. As an important variable in population health studies ethnicity is most studied as a concern in societies with larger ethnic minorities. For example, whereas the US public policy on inequities has focused on racial inequalities, the UK government has focused on disparities in geography and socioeconomic status (Exworthy et al., 2006). South Africa is another more extreme example in which apartheid and deliberate inequalities have had profound effects on the majority non-white populations, and race is an important issue. Even years after the establishment of a democratic government, discrimination persists and health inequalities are worsening (Geiger, 2003; Sanders and Chopra, 2006). However, in other countries these same racial inequalities may exist, but receive less attention. For example, Australia is described as an egalitarian country when statistics are considered across the whole population (Wilkinson, 2005). However, Australia includes an indigenous population with very poor health status. Indigenous life expectation is 17 years lower than for other Australians; infant mortality is three times higher; and death rates for Indigenous Australians are twice as high across all age groups (Human Rights and Equal Opportunity Commission, 2008). Although for the general population in Australia, life expectancy is increasing rapidly, health inequality has remained static or continued to grow. Indigenous peoples' self-assessed health status also shows that the percentage of Indigenous respondents assessing their health as 'fair/ poor' rose from 17.5 to 23.3 percent. Correspondingly, there was no increase in the number who assessed their health as 'excellent/very good' or reported reductions in smoking or alcohol consumption. The high mortality rate of Aboriginal people does not impact on the generally low mortality of the Australian population as a whole and the most attention to the care of Aboriginal peoples is found in the health policy, health promotion or other health professional literature (e.g., Jamieson et al., 2007). Similarly the aboriginal Inuit people of Canada also have problems that deserve serious consideration but may be missed in population approaches (e.g., Ho et al., 2006).

Gendered inequalities

In many epidemiological studies, men were the primary object of study. When women were included, the data were often aggregated. MacIntyre and Hunt (1997) were concerned to point out that simply including women in this way does not take into account the different distribution of paid work and domestic roles of men and women, and their very different material and social experiences. Most of our social life is deeply structured on the basis of gender so that gender is ubiquitous and therefore taken for granted. It may be for this very reason that reasons for gender differences are not often discussed in health related research. The general understanding that women live longer than men but have more illnesses in their lifetime has often been an unexamined assumption in epidemiological research. This is despite more complex evidence that shows that these sorts of differences are subject to historical, material and cultural changes. MacIntyre and Hunt suggest that our knowledge about the relationships between socioeconomic status and health would be enhanced by taking gendered differences more seriously.

In general, the evidence drawn upon for MacIntyre and Hunt's (1997) review shows that there are differences in the socioeconomic status and mortality gradient between men and women. Measures of education, income, occupation and area deprivation in the US, Britain, France, Hungary, Norway and Denmark showed that the gradient is more likely to be steeper for men (see Figure 3.3 for an example). There are some differences between the gradients for men and women when the cause of mortality is considered. Taken together these differences support the notion that the structure of women's and men's lives includes different exposures and risks. There are some notable differences when additional aspects of social status are taken into account. For example, a study in Finland found the steeper gradient for men, but only for married persons. Among single, widowed or divorced women the mortality gradient was as steep for women as for men. Tsuchiya and Williams (2005) raise the issue of men's excess mortality and suggest that the current distribution of health in most countries does not give men a 'fair innings'. However, in considering the broader social context with its many levels of inequality they conclude that these are questions about general well being that remain unresolved.

In regard to morbidity, an even more complex picture emerges. There are few consistent differences in class related gradients on various illness measures between men and women. Popay et al. (1993) suggest that women

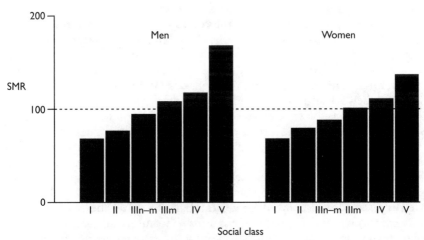

Figure 3.3 Standardized mortality ratios (SMRs) for men aged 20–64 and women aged 20–59, by occupational class around the 1981 census, Great Britain

Source: From Macintyre and Hunt, 1997; reproduced by permission of Sage Publications Ltd.

.report more illnesses in general, not across a gradient but because they are more likely to occupy the lower social positions that are related to higher rates of ill health. For women in the same occupational positions as men, the findings show complex differences. Across a number of studies, the results for men and women differ according to the illness measured, so that for some illnesses women do not reflect the gradient found more regularly among men. For example, the Whitehall II study (Marmot and Davey Smith, 1997) found that higher grade women had more sickness days than the grade below them. These highest grade women also smoked more, which is different to the men for whom the inverse gradient between smoking and grade was continuous. Several other studies have reported similar results for women in high status jobs (MacIntyre and Hunt, 1997) suggesting that these women have a different experience and perhaps more stressors than men. Other evidence in regard to CHD (Brezinka and Kittel, 1996) demonstrates the interaction of another set of circumstances for working class women. Although the incidence of CHD remains lower for women, the relationship between SES and CHD is steeper for women: women of lower SES are more likely to die from CHD. At the same time, evidence shows that work and family combined increases women's risk of heart disease. Research has also shown that, women as a group are treated differently in health care settings in regard to CHD. In Britain, women with suspected CHD, as well as with CHD documented by MI or coronary angiography, have been shown to have less access to major diagnostic and treatment procedures (Brezinka and Kittel, 1996). In the US, 4 percent of abnormal radionuclide scans were referred for cardiac catheterization compared to 40 percent for men (Rodin and Ickovics, 1990).

Once we begin enquiring into the results of large population studies by comparing results for different groups and taking into account more complex interactions, many assumptions about group differences or similarities, and about the universal operation of standardized variables come up for questioning. The gendered segregation of employment including paid work, housework and care giving must be considered when we are thinking about the effects of social status on health for both sexes. Some recent studies have enquired into these relationships. For example, Borrell et al. (2004) found that among men, part of the association between social class positions and health was accounted for by working conditions and job insecurity. Among women, the association between the occupational class positions and health was substantially explained by working conditions as well as material well being at home and their amount of household labour. In regard to women and social status, it has become clear that the measures of socioeconomic status developed in research with men do not apply in the same way. More recent studies in other countries have enquired into these differences (Artazcoz et al., 2004; Denton et al., 2004). Their findings raise important questions about the different material, social and psychological meanings for men and women of variables like education, income, wealth, housing and work. This is without considering the interactions of gender and ethnicity which is another whole area of consideration and research that we must note and leave aside for now. This is only for reasons of space, not because the interplay of gender and ethnicity does not have very important consequences for health in different societies.

Explanations for social inequalities in health

Understanding the gradient

There are two unequivocal understandings raised by the wealth of support for the relationship between social inequalities and health outcomes. First, that the observed relationship is on a gradient. It is not just about the differences that poverty makes to health (although these are manifest). It is about differences in social status and health at every level of society and these differences may be observed among wealthy as well as poor people. Second, that the health differences are relative to the status of those in the same society or group, not to absolute levels of material wealth. These understandings together do not mean that we should direct interventions towards wealthy people like Oscar contenders. Rather, they have major implications for public health, health promotion and social policies because they reveal the importance of psychosocial factors in promoting health for all. In addition, this evidence points us away from a focus on the responsibility of individuals for their health, towards a concern with whole societies.

However, we need a greater understanding of how this relationship works. How does relative status work to produce such fine grained differences in biological outcomes? What exactly is it about social life that impacts on the body, and what are the links between social life and disease? Epidemiological evidence has provided valuable demonstrations of the regularities between social position and health outcomes. However, these broad population-based approaches are not so useful at generating explanations. For that we need theories about how social life affects physical health. These under-standings are at the crux of the issue today. Despite a great deal of interest in these questions and growing acceptance by policymakers and governments that inequalities are an important aspect of health, the mechanisms and relationships are still not well understood, and there is a need for ongoing consideration and research. Many possibilities have been suggested, some have been abandoned and some are being vigorously pursued. There are some areas of keen contention between researchers, health workers and social policy analysts.

Health related behaviours

One of the first and obvious explanations of the data was that behaviours, such as diet, smoking, condom use or exercise that directly affect health outcomes, are also closely related to social class. The best example for this argument is smoking, since there is little doubt about the deleterious effects of smoking on physical health. In addition, there is a great deal of evidence to show that people of lower incomes, lower social class, lower occupational grades or lower education, are more likely to smoke (e.g., Pugh et al., 1991; Chamberlain, 1997). There have been many investigations into the reasons for this relationship leading to research showing that health related behaviours are not simply a matter of individual understanding and decision making. Rather, behaviour is an integral part of daily social life. For example, Chamberlain and O'Neill (1998) noted that differences in accounts of the meanings of smoking and health, understandings of personal control over health, and reasons for smoking are embedded in differences in daily social and cultural life. Crossley (2000a) has pointed to the historical nature of behaviours such as condom use, and described the ways in which these behaviours are embedded in an unconsciously enacted 'cultural psyche'.

The chief aim of work from an epidemiological perspective is to separate causal factors. This approach has been used to discount the suggestion that health related behaviour explains the gradient by statistically controlling for smoking. The Whitehall studies controlled for smoking carefully since it is a risk factor for CHD. In both the first Whitehall study and a follow up, Whitehall II (which included women and considered more social and behavioural factors), there were certainly differences across the grades in smoking as expected: lower grade employees were more likely to smoke. However, the grade differences in smoking did not account for differences by grade in mortality, even from smoking related diseases (Marmot and Davey Smith, 1997). Furthermore, from Whitehall II comes the information that exercise patterns and healthy diets were also negatively related to occupational grade but, if controlled for in the same way, did not affect the relationship between occupational status and mortality.

These statistical techniques may be turned around to show that social status explains a good portion of smoking related deaths. Blakely et al. (2004) showed that taking account of socioeconomic position (measured by both neighbourhood level deprivation and individual socioeconomic status) reduced the association of smoking and mortality by 26 percent for men and 19 percent for women. Barnett et al. (2005) studied the effects of growing inequalities between Māori and non-Māori in New Zealand from 1981 to 1996 to show that communities which experienced increased inequality also had higher smoking rates for Māori (especially for women). Blakely and colleagues (2006) have also examined the relative effects of ethnicity, socio-economic status and smoking on mortality using census data and mortality records for 45–74 year-olds. They concluded that 'the contribution of socioeconomic position to ethnic disparities in mortality in New Zealand was substantially greater than that of smoking' and that 'tackling SES disparities between ethnic groups stands out as an important strategy to reduce ethnic inequalities in mortality' (p. 50). Similar findings in the UK had led

Wilkinson to write in 1999, 'the well known behavioural risk factors left most of the social gradient in health unexplained' (p. 48). This does not mean that health related behaviours are unimportant. It does mean that there are underlying social factors contributing to health behaviours that we still do not understand well. Understanding more about the forces underlying the gradient effect will also help us to understand the intertwining of risky health behaviours, social status, ethnicity and health outcomes.

Health care inequities

Inequalities in health care have also been considered as a serious issue. In many areas of health care including access to all medical services, receipt of public health services such as vaccinations and uptake of health promotion education, there is a wealth of evidence regarding inequalities, even in countries with universal state provision of health care. There is considerable evidence that patients are treated inequitably in health care settings according to their race, ethnicity or social status. In the US, where there is a great deal of concern and interest in such inequities, the Institute of Medicine has published a report entitled, *Unequal Treatment: Confronting Racial and Ethnic Disparities in Health Care* (Smedley et al., 2003). The report concluded that 'patients of color tend to receive a lower quality of health care than white patients and that these disparities exact a significant toll on individuals, families and communities' (Smedley, 2006, p. 539). Within the same report Byrd and Clayton (2003) note a further 600 scientific publications that document racial and ethnic disparities in health care. Geiger (2003) has reviewed much of this evidence to demonstrate disparities of treatment and outcomes between African American, Hispanic, Native American and Asian people compared with white people, across general medical and surgical care as well as coronary artery diseases, cancers, stroke, renal diseases and HIV/AIDS. Geiger notes that there is also evidence for disparities in other illness contexts and in other countries such as South Africa, Australia, Canada, France, Israel and the UK. In New Zealand, evidence for racial disparities comes from differences between mortality rates for amenable diseases, that is diseases such as CHD for which early deaths are preventable. Sporle et al. (2002) showed that overall Māori are 5.3 times more likely to die of a cause that is amenable to intervention than non-Māori. These rates increase across the occupational class gradient, but, controlling for occupation only reduces this ratio to 4.8. So, other factors are also contributing to these disparities.

Byrd and Clayton (2003) point to contemporary evidence suggesting that as well as socioeconomic differences (which directly contribute to inadequate access to health care where there is no universal provision), other important factors include racial, ethnic, class and gender bias, and direct and indirect discrimination. The sources of such bias and discrimination include racism, biased clinical decision making, a health system structured on the basis of race, ethnicity and class, and access barriers caused by shortages of minority providers. Again, there is a great deal of evidence, particularly from ethnographic studies in disciplines such as psychology and anthropology, and from countries across the world, for the operation of these deep-seated biases among dominant groups (McCreanor and Nairn, 2002; Geiger, 2003; Good et al., 2003).

Despite the importance of eliminating these unjust disparities, they are not sufficient to explain the relationship between social status and health. This is largely because medical care and individually focused health promotion interventions are not the most important contributers to health outcomes, and a focus on health care systems has very limited potential to reduce health disparities (Smedley, 2006). Although, there was an emphasis on the provision of public health services following World War II, followed by an emphasis on lifestyle factors in the 1970s, since the 1980s public health researchers have understood that medical services are not the major contributor to population health (Wilkinson, 1999).

Marmot (2004) dismisses health care as having any direct explanatory power. He points to mounting epidemiological evidence since the 1970s for the very low impact of medical intervention and the corresponding awareness of the importance of social conditions. Wilkinson (2005) has also carefully considered this explanation. He notes that the effects of who gets medical care are certainly observable (as in Sporle and colleagues' data above), but they are dwarfed by differences in who actually contracts the illnesses. Marmot (1999) provides a very good example of how individual risk factors (i.e., the precursors to getting the disease) are related to rates of mortality from CHD, but do not explain the gradient. Marmot shows graphically how the social gradient shows up *within* levels of plasma cholesterol, which is a risk factor for CHD. Whitehall men in the highest occupational level have the lowest CHD mortality rate as we know. In addition, the lowest rates of cholesterol levels were among the administrators, with increasing rates of high cholesterol levels across the occupational grades. Those in 'other occupations' had the highest rates of cholesterol levels. The predisposition to illness such as CHD is already in place according to social status.

Researchers and policy analysts in the area of health care disparities themselves seem to agree that the basis of inequalities is not medical care or lifestyle change, but the relations produced by differences in race, ethnicity, class, culture, socioeconomic status and gender (Byrd and Clayton, 2003; Smedley, 2006). Given these understandings, it seems more useful to see health care disparities, not as an explanation, but as a symptom of the broader social inequalities that are affecting health. In writing about the need to tackle growing inequalities and the problems of poverty in developing countries, Feachem (2000) is sceptical about the efficacy of provision of health services to the poor as a solution. He notes the wealth of evidence showing that public subsidies for health, education, water or food, are routinely captured by the non-poor, especially the middle class. We have also seen examples of this in campaigns for lifestyle change in developed countries: changes in behaviours such as smoking, diet or exercise tend to be taken up mainly by those who are already well off. Understandings of the broader issues of social inequalities should be used to assist our understandings of the fundamental nature and perpetuation of health care inequalities.

Psychosocial and biological pathways

Since working on the Whitehall studies and other large scale studies of health in Britain, both Richard Wilkinson and Michael Marmot have shifted their attention from the material and medical causes of disease to explanations for the striking relationships between psychosocial factors and population health that have emerged from the data. Both have expressed their surprise at the direction that their findings have taken them, but both have used a wide range of evidence to develop theses about the importance of social and economic inequalities, and of psychosocial factors as an explanation for the effects on population health. Marmot (2004, 2006) has focused his most recent musings on the fundamental importance of the gradient in health inequalities and what he terms the 'status syndrome'. Wilkinson (1999, 2005) has focused on inequalities in the steepness of the gradient between countries, and evidence that shows that less egalitarian societies are worse for the health of the whole population. Both draw on very similar ideas and on a great deal of evidence in common, although there are some differences. Both argue for the importance of changes in population health for changes in individual health outcomes. Since Wilkinson has developed the most coherent thesis, I will begin with a brief account of his ideas along with some of the additional understandings that Marmot brings in from his own work.

Wilkinson's most recent explanations are described in his book, *The Impact of Inequality* (2005) and this description is based on that work. After considering the evidence for the relationship between inequalities of income between countries or states and their mortality rates or other health indices, Wilkinson has concluded that more egalitarian societies have healthier populations. His explanation for the effect of income inequality on the health of a whole population follows a clearly described pathway which implicates social relations and psychosocial factors. First, wider income inequalities reflect poorer social relations. Second, poorer social relations are related to health through three main psychosocial risk factors that have been shown to affect health. Third, these factors can be linked to other psychological risks to well being. Fourth, these factors are all seen as sources of chronic stress which directly affects physical health through hormonal activity.

In regard to poorer social relations, Wilkinson contends that income has been useful as a measure of inequality across countries, but must be seen as related to other aspects of social life. To support this he draws on a wide range of evidence which shows that higher income inequalities, racial inequalities and health inequalities are related to more conflict, homicide, violent crime and racism, and less trust and community involvement. He also notes evidence that in countries with more equality for women or between ethnic groups, health is better for men and women, for blacks and .whites. All of these variables are seen to reflect underlying variations in the quality of social relationships in a country or state.

Poor quality social relations are related to poor population health through three main psychosocial pathways: social status, social support, and early emotional and social development. Wilkinson draws on a great deal of psychological theory and evidence to show that these three factors are negatively affected by unequal social relations. Furthermore, they are the three most potent psychosocial factors that have been reliably shown to affect health. Wilkinson also draws on an overarching theoretical construct, social insecurity or anxiety (he uses both terms), to suggest that these three factors are part of a fundamental need for social approval that underpins the functioning of our social relations.

If things are going badly for a person's social status, social support and childhood development, other evidence suggests that this will affect important psychological outcomes such as sense of control, self-esteem, depression and hostility. Of course, all these are known to be related to physical health. In addition, Wilkinson suggests the workings of shame, a complex social emotion, are important in making these links.

Before moving on to the biological pathways, for which both Wilkinson and Marmot draw on similar explanations and evidence, I will note Marmot's contributions to this field, chiefly from his book of the same period, *The Status Syndrome* (1994). As the title suggests, Marmot builds his explanation for the connection between socioeconomic status and health around the central importance of social standing. In particular, he is concerned with the effects of our relative position to others in our society. He also provides evidence of links between low status and poor social relations reflected in violence. Like Wilkinson, he draws on the rich evidence for the importance of social support (including family, childhood experience, social relations outside the family, social networks and social capital), the work environment and control at work (to which his own work has contributed), and sense of control in general. In addition, Marmot suggests that socioeconomic status contributes to people's ability to participate in their society. This is an important point in explaining the gradient and the relative nature of deprivation. If a person in a developed country has food, clothes, water and an indoor bathroom, why might they still be sicker than a poor person in a society with fewer of these basic needs? Marmot reasons that the inability to go on a holiday, pursue a hobby or buy new clothes for a child is not absolute poverty but it is very real deprivation because it reflects an inability to participate in one's own society. Such participation is essential for health.

Participation is also conceivably related to notions of the important effects of social insecurity and shame.

Both authors suggest that the psychological effects of the social factors result in chronic stress. Wilkinson in particular provides evidence that low social status, lack of friends and childhood stress are all associated with raised basal cortisol levels, which are used as a measure of the body's stress reactions. A recent review of the stressors affecting cortisol responses suggests that uncontrollable threats to self-esteem and social status are the most important (Dickerson and Kemeny, 2005). Increased cortisol production has been linked to insulin resistance, raised blood sugar, raised blood pressure and high cholesterol. This human evidence is linked to studies with wild baboons, in which low status baboons (who don't smoke, eat hamburgers or fail to keep doctor's appointments, as Marmot puts it) have higher basal cortisol levels than higher status baboons (who don't have gym membership or read health information). The lower the baboon's rank, the higher the basal cortisol and the lower the level of HDL cholesterol (low levels are associated with increased risk of heart disease). This finding was reflected in the Whitehall II studies in which the lower the rank, the lower the HDL cortisol. Further evidence is also provided by experimental studies with Macacque monkeys in which diet and all living conditions were controlled. These studies showed that given a high fat diet, the higher the rank of the animal, the less likely it was to build up cholesterol-rich placques in blood vessels. And these effects could be changed by manipulating the status of the animal. Other effects of social life among monkeys have also been found for important hormones such as serotonin and dopamine, linked to depression and drug use in humans.

Marmot's explanations focus on the effects of social status as a stressor, particularly in regard to low status citizens who are in jobs in which they have little personal control or who are unable to fully participate in society. Wilkinson's thesis adds the explanation that in a more hierarchical society, people may be more aware of status, more conscious of threats to their status and more anxious about potential change (such as through unemployment or falling behind). Thus, both those at the lower end of society (who bear the brunt) but even those in higher positions (like Oscar nominees) are subject to increased social anxiety and stress.

Neo-materialist and structural explanations

An important opposing set of explanations is suggested by the 'neo-materialist interpretation' of the data (Lynch et al., 2000). This says that health inequalities result from exposures to material causes of ill health. For example, in 1997, Marmot and Davey Smith argued that occupational grade may be a proxy for salary which in turn relates to material conditions outside work. They related the Whitehall findings to links between deprivation and mortality found in geographically-based studies. In the UK, rating neighbourhoods along a continuum of 'deprivation' according to unemployment, overcrowding, housing and car ownership levels shows that there is a strong relationship between level of deprivation and mortality across the whole index (i.e., on a gradient). Hence, income inequality is seen as just one aspect of material conditions such as environment, education, food, health services, housing that all cluster together (i.e., if you have less education, you have lower income, poorer housing, a worse environment, etc.) and reflect differences in individual access to this wide range of resources. This understanding is based on known links to health through micro-organisms and to disease risks from differing conditions such as housing and the environment (Kaplan et al., 1996). For instance, low quality housing is associated with higher rates of respiratory disease, and air pollution levels in different cities are associated with different levels of mortality (Carroll et al., 1996).

The neo-materialist conceptualization is based on the recognition that although one adverse physical event may have a small effect, the clustering of adverse factors has a cumulative effect on health. Thus, people at different levels in a hierarchical society are subject to different clusters of adversity. People are also seen as generally subject to a range of problems or benefits that accrue to different groups, right across their lifecourse. These exposures and experiences accumulate and show up in patterns of mortality for different social groups. The evidence and explanation for these effects tends to come from the low end of the social scale and focus on the more intuitively understood effects of poverty. Thus, Carroll and colleagues (1996) describe an example of potential life course clustering: a baby born to a lower-SES mother is more likely to register low birth weight and growing up in a low-SES household is more likely to experience family instability, poor diet, damp and overcrowding, and poorer education. As an adolescent, the child is more likely to experience family strife, smoke cigarettes, leave school early, and experience unemployment and/or low paid insecure work. As an adult she or he is more likely to work in an arduous, hazardous job, suffer financial insecurity, more stress and less happiness, with less control over her or his life. Once retired she or he is unlikely to have an occupational pension and more likely to have poorer clothing, heating and diet, and greater social isolation. Thus, across a lifetime, such an accumulation of factors could result in considerable disadvantage, compared to a person of higher status who has none of these experiences. Authors who support this view also draw on evidence to show that changes in a group's economic situation can improve their health, such as evidence for the improvements in different countries in birth weight for children whose mothers received some form of income supplement (Carroll et al., 1996). It should also be noted here, that Davey Smith et al. (1997) used longitudinal data from Scottish men to show the lifetime effects of childhood disadvantage. Men from working class families who subsequently went to university and took up middle class occupations were still more likely to die earlier from CHD. It turns out that social class in early life and subsequent social status in adulthood both independently predict poor health or early mortality in later life.

The important point of the accumulation of disadvantage is that it is used to support the neo-materialist argument for structural causes of ill health. That is, unequal income distribution is one result of historical, cultural and political economic processes that have structured society in its present form (Lynch et al., 2000). It is a 'top–down' explanation in that the structure of society is assumed to be in place before the individuals who fill its places. It is related to investments in health related infrastructure or sharing of resources by the state, and accordingly is amenable to intervention particularly at state level. The political import of the argument, then, is that interventions at the level of individual psychosocial variables such as social support, or of community level variables such as social capital, are not helpful. They have the effect of placing responsibility for poor health and for change on those individuals and communities with the least resources, and taking the responsibility away from the state or the whole of society. Notice that, according to the lifecourse example above, the neo-materialist argument does not discount the effect of psychosocial factors. However, the focus is on the amenable aspects of the clustering of disadvantage from a structural perspective. This is a focus on the political and economic structure of society, and the amenable effects of poorer material conditions. Lynch et al. (2000) argue for the need for practical investments in public health interventions such as redistribution of income and the development of public health infrastructure which includes good housing, living and working conditions made available for all.

The neo-materialist position takes into account material needs that still exist in developed countries but in this regard tends to focus on broad inequalities between the wealthy and the poor. The material effects of very poor housing and a dangerous environment are important to health and there is no doubt that, like smoking and obesity, which are also related to deprivation, they are important issues which deserve intervention in their own right. However, it does not contribute an explanation for the relationship between deprivation and health across a gradient. It fails to explain the health differences among quite well off people and the population effects of widening inequalities. Some researchers have taken up oppositional neo-materialist or psychosocial positions and many disputes about the interpretation of epidemiological data, and what counts as main effect or control variables, have been conducted on these grounds (e.g., Adler, 2006).

Researchers on both sides of the debate ostensibly argue for the same outcome: a reduction of social and economic inequalities which will demonstrably lead to a reduction in health inequalities and resulting better health for all. All public health researchers are committed to finding solutions that will lead to effective intervention and health promotion. At bottom, the disputes about interpretation of research findings are about where the focus of these interventions should lie. Psychosocial explanations have been taken up enthusiastically by health promoters with a 'communitarian' approach. This approach focuses on community development and participation by community members in health promotion activities (more about this later). From this applied perspective, the development of constructs like social capital and trust among members of neighbourhoods and suburbs has seemed like an appealing way to develop community health. Proponents of the neo-materialist approach see the dangers in these approaches: dangers of holding poor people responsible for developing their own resources, while allowing governments to neglect the distribution of material resources that will reduce inequalities. These disputes are important because they keep the focus of all public health research keenly on the objective of improving population health. At the same time the debates highlight the need to continue to develop our understandings of the relationship between social and health inequalities so that policies and interventions may be more effective in the future.

Developing effective interventions

Many theorists and researchers are working toward a reconciliation of psychosocial and material understandings. The lifecourse approach has been recognized as having a great deal of potential to explain the long-term and structured experiences of people, while including both psychosocial and material effects on health together. Following a government sponsored inquiry in the UK, Acheson (1998) suggested that lifestyle factors, social networks, working conditions and other determinants of health are unequally stratified by social position and act together as 'layers of influence' to determine individual health outcomes. Researchers following this line suggest a turn to considering the complex interactions between material, social and individual circumstances across time (e.g., Carroll et al., 1996; MacIntyre and Hunt, 1997; Adler, 2006). Singh-Manoux and Marmot (2005) have sought to bring together the neo-materialist/structural and psychosocial explanations for social inequalities in health by suggesting four key areas that theoretically link social structure and environment to health. The main focus of research in this area remains on using epidemiological methods, with increasingly sophisticated analytic techniques to investigate the layered and prospective measures needed to account for time, individual differences in gender, ethnicity and income, wider social factors, and the environment. These approaches have shown us the complexity of the threads that contribute to health differentials, but they are not so helpful at providing explanations (and in fact tend to create the current divisions and debates). The results still tend to demonstrate linear relationships and Exworthy et al. (2006) have talked about the difficulties of translating this sort of evidence into practice: 'In sum, much of the evidence to date has emphasized description, with relatively little attention to theories and models of causation' (p. 82).

Summary

There is strong support for the observation, largely from epidemiological evidence, that inequalities in SES are related to health across a gradient. Particular groupings in society, such as ethnicity, also demonstrate inequalities in health outcomes, beyond those related to other markers of social status such as income and occupation. There are ongoing controversies in the academic literature about the interpretation of these findings. The basis of these controversies is how our understandings of the effects will translate into public policy and health promotion interventions that will be useful and not damaging to people who already suffer poorer health. Although there are presently moves to integrate the competing explanations in regard to practical interventions, this work remains problematic while our explanations remain unclear.

Inequalities in health are a very clear example of a health issue in which we need better explanations for empirical observations. This situation highlights the need for the use of theoretical approaches that will be helpful in developing explanations for the complexities of social life, material life and health. The employment of good theory will develop explanation and point to alternative methodologies to develop an understanding of the empirical observations of regularities and associations in populations. In the next chapter, I will develop the importance of theory in health promotion more broadly. In Chapter 4, this discussion will move on to alternative methodological approaches that provide us with tools to enquire into and develop these understandings.

Further reading

1 I recommend the most recent books by Marmot and Wilkinson as cited above (as well as other work by these influential authors):
Marmot, M.G. (2004) *The Status Syndrome: How Social Standing Affects Our Health and Longevity*. New York: Henry Holt.
Wilkinson, R.G. (2005) *The Impact of Inequality: How to Make Sick Societies Healthier*. London: Routledge.
2 For comments by critics of the psychosocial approach to understanding inequalities apparently propounded by Marmot and Wilkinson see:
Lynch, J.W., Davey Smith, G., Kaplan, G.A. and House, J.S. (2000) Income inequality and mortality: importance to health of individual income, psychosocial environment, or material conditions, *British Medical Journal*, 320(29 April), 1200–4.
Lynch, J., Harper, S. and Davey Smith, G. (2003) Commentary: plugging leaks and repelling boarders – where to next for the SS income inequality? *International Journal of Epidemiology*, 32(6), 1029–36.

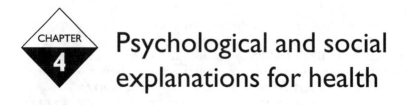

Psychological and social explanations for health

Introduction

This chapter describes theoretical approaches to the point made in Chapter 1 that health behaviour is socially oriented. I will outline some of the key theoretical explanations of this position which is underscored by the need for good theory. We need theory because it provides explanations for health, health behaviours and the importance of social life in health. All explanations are theory but too often these explanations are taken for granted and unexamined. Explicitly described theory that is available for critique and testing is the basis of reflexive practice. Theory used reflexively is practical and ethical. Having coherent testable explanations for phenomena will help us to develop practices and interventions that work and avoid doing harm.

Need for theory

When we observe phenomena in the world we leap to explanations. As shown in the last chapter, there is compelling data from epidemiological research that seems to clearly point to a relationship between social status and health outcomes. These data do not provide any explanation for these links, although explanations have been suggested. The health inequalities literature shows that when we start with observation quite fierce controversies about how to explain or use these observations can develop. We need good theory to guide our ongoing understanding and explanation of the basis of such phenomena. In particular we often want to explain causality. Does social status actually cause ill health? And what are the mechanisms for this? Theory provides coherently structured explanations for what can be a confusing diversity of observations and insights.

Any explanation is a theory. Some theories are more carefully thought out than others. We all have theories about how things work in the world, about why some people have more resources than others, and why some people get sicker than others. We have many theories about how to keep ourselves healthy and what health means. Many of these theories involve implicit assumptions and taken for granted knowledge. Others have been learned in a more overt way from textbooks and scholarly papers. A great deal of health promotion work happens somewhere in between the two. There are many well thought out and overtly scrutinized theories to explain the social aspects of health, but there is also a great deal of activity based on poorly examined assumptions about the basis of health. To guide understandings of the basis of health issues, to understand the complexities of health related behaviour, and to include insights into the social structures that affect health, and to be critical of our own assumptions, we need to draw on good theories.

What is a good theory? There is a wealth of theory available to explain health and health behaviours. The most important criteria for a theory's usefulness is that it is acknowledged, well described and thus available for scrutiny. If we are able to describe our explanations in a coherent fashion, then we are also able to discuss them with others, acknowledge critique and test their efficacy in application. In an applied field like health promotion this efficacy, that is the theory's ability to explain our observations and fit with new observations, is an important aspect of its use. The acknowledgement and ongoing critique of the theories that we use is a critical aspect of reflexive practice.

Theory enables us to be reflexive about our activities and in this way, the use of theory is supremely practical. There are two very practical aspects to the use of explicit theory in health promotion. First, it is very important that we use understandings that make sense and fit together (i.e., are coherent). If health promotion efforts are based on faulty thinking and false understandings of the basis of health and health behaviour, then they simply will not work. Second, and further to this, they may do harm. Without clear understandings of the reasons behind our actions and the wider web of related relationships, some health promotion actions may have unintended consequences. For example, in defining a health issue, it is important to understand the social consequences of the theories used to decide what the issue is. Whaley (2003) has described how the cultural heritage of racism continues to colour the interpretation of epidemiological data showing poorer health for African Americans. Health promotion practice influenced by unacknowledged theories of racial inferiority focuses on individual failings, rather than on the sociocultural practices of racism that maintain disadvantage. Research on an issue based on a particular theoretical approach may also be detrimental. Public health researchers, concerned about the health of babies born to disadvantaged parents have focused on the 'problem' of adolescent motherhood in suggesting the causes of poor outcomes for babies. This construction of teenage mothers as a problem, which has been taken up uncritically by the media, works to stigmatize young mothers, rather than to value their parenting and focus on the social and structural basis of their babies' disadvantage. In regard to intervention practice itself, an example of what seems like a 'good idea' comes from some early AIDS prevention campaigns. These were based on messages designed to invoke fear of the consequences of unprotected sex (such as 'grim reaper' television advertisements). Such messages were based on assumptions that if people were afraid of the consequences they would change their behaviour. However, the ads were found to be so frightening that many people just switched them off. Cognitive psychological theories explain that if we do not know how to deal with a threat, then denial is the best coping mechanism. Good theory is an ethical requirement for any stage of health promotion work from issue definition through research to intervention.

Which theory?

Choosing a theoretical approach does not suggest that we may select an explanation to fit all situations. In a field of applied science, such as health promotion, there are many different aspects of health to be considered and many different approaches to theory available for us to draw on to explain health phenomena. As we have seen in Chapter 2, health psychologists working in health promotion may be involved in research and practice related to issues ranging from implications for health policy, through community projects, to considerations of individual adjustment to illness. This means that there are many possible theoretical explanations for the aspects of health that we are concerned with. Stam (2000) makes the case for the importance of theory for social scientists of any discipline across all of these practices, and moreover, of the importance of a reflexive approach to choosing theory. He says:

> I want to make the case that theory is not a luxury or what one does after a hard day of collecting data. On the contrary, it is one of the most crucial steps of our entry into the world of health, disease and illness precisely because it establishes nothing less than our political, epistemological and moral grounding. It also establishes our responsibility as professionals who intervene in the lives of others even if done at the level of research.
>
> (p. 276)

Stam's is a call for a reflexive approach to theorizing health and illness that acknowledges the professional position and personal responsibility of health psychologists. If we unpack his focus on 'political, epistemological and moral grounding' we have a good basis for considering theories of health.

Epistemology

Our approach to theorizing health establishes the epistemological basis of our knowledge of health and health related behaviours. Epistemology involves the understanding of knowledge itself, how knowledge is produced, and the status of knowledge. It is important that we are aware of how our knowledge has been produced and the role of that knowledge in our practice. A reflexive approach to theory takes into account the basis of the knowledge produced by the 'scientific knower' and also the personal and social position of the 'knower' and the use of that knowledge.

Political and moral values

Understanding the political and moral basis of health promotion research and practice opens the way for a consideration of theory on this basis. Choosing theory means deciding which political and moral values we will pursue in our practice within the community in which we also recognize ourselves as active participants (not impartial outsiders).

Thus, attention to epistemology and values in choosing theoretical approaches to health also means recognizing our position as professionals who are members (not objective outsiders) of the social order in which we are working. In the following sections, I will outline some theories that have been used in health promotion. These are grouped according to a broad epistemological basis and accompanied by a discussion of the values implied by each approach. These groups also reflect a shift along a continuum of epistemological concern from individual experience and behaviour to the social and structural basis of health. We will see that the place of the values embedded in these approaches also shift from the unacknowledged 'value free' approach to concerted political involvement. The theoretical orientations grouped together here have been labelled (as broadly descriptive and not to be regarded as definitive): positivist, interpretivist, social constructionist, social and critical social. In addition, I have included a discussion of clashing epistemologies and an emerging participatory epistemology as themes particularly relevant to health promotion practice.

Predicting behaviour (neo-positivism)

Theoretical approaches in psychology have long been dominated by versions of positivism or logical positivism. Positivist theorizing (developed from early empiricism) is based on an objectivist epistemology which holds that reality exists apart from any consciousness and knowledge is gained through observation. Owing to the emphasis on the observed effects of causal relations in the world, this approach eschews formal theory development. Epidemiological research is a good example of a neo-positivist approach, in which observations of large groups of people are made (often through surveys) and inferential statistics used to assess relationships between variables in the population. Psychologists use both survey and experimental methods to generate findings (based on aggregated data and statistical inference) about the relationships of psychosocial variables to health or health related behaviour among groups of people. It is too simple to claim that this sort of psychological research is pure positivism. Psychology has many branches and there are many variants of neo-positivism, such as the hypothetico-deductive model used by cognitive social psychologists, in which hypotheses are tested with the aim of refuting theoretical propositions. Social cognitive models of behaviour provide relevant examples of the application of neo-positivist theorizing about health.

Social cognitive models

To explain health related behaviour, health psychologists have lately drawn heavily upon social cognitive models of behaviour. These theoretical models are designed to generate hypotheses for testing and provide specific targets for intervention. That is, the definition of specific cognitions such as beliefs and attitudes, provide health promoters with aspects of people's thinking that may be changed through counselling, education programmes or media campaigns. There are several versions of social cognitive theories that have been used in health promotion work. These are summarized in texts such as Bennett and Murphy (1997). Bandura's (1986) social learning theory may be seen as a precursor and basis for this sort of theorizing, and Bandura's work remains the most theoretically developed work in this area. In particular his concepts of self-efficacy and learning through social modelling have been very influential in developing health promotion interventions. To provide brief examples of other popular models I have chosen two: the health belief model; and the theory of planned behaviour.

Health belief model

This popular model for health promotion work was developed by Becker in the 1970s (Bennett and Murphy, 1997). This model suggests that people make decisions about health related behaviour, such as using a condom, engaging in exercise, or attending breast screening, based on two kinds of appraisals: beliefs about the threat of illness (e.g., I could get breast cancer: cancer is a potentially fatal illness) and beliefs about the behaviour itself (e.g., breast screening will protect me: I can keep an appointment for screening). In addition to these four beliefs (labelled: perceived susceptibility, perceived severity, perceived benefits and perceived barriers) an additional factor is external cues to action (such as a doctor's recommendation). Accordingly, a campaign to increase breast screening behaviour based on this model would need to consider and target all five cognitions in some way.

Theory of planned behaviour

There is no explanation in the health belief model of how the different beliefs work together or actually affect behaviour, so each of the five variables is seen as independently contributing somehow to the behavioural decision. In a more sophisticated model including similar variables, Ajzen and Fishbein developed attitudinal theories which suggest that the formation of cognitive intentions is the precursor to behaviour. Their theory of planned behaviour (Bennett and Murphy, 1997) suggests that attitudes, subjective norms (social norms as perceived by the individual) and perceptions of one's ability to perform the behaviour, together predict these intentions. Intentions, along with perceived behavioural control, will in turn predict whether a person engages in the behaviour itself.

This theory has been well researched in many health related areas such as condom use, healthy eating, seat belt wearing and not smoking with some initially encouraging results. However, the weakest relationship remains that between intentions and behaviour. This suggests that many other environmental factors are influencing people's behaviour, despite their stated intentions. For example, the relationship between intentions to use condoms and actual use has been shown to be much weaker for women than for men. This is in accord with qualitative studies that have revealed women's lack of power in the sexual relationship (Bennett and Murphy, 1997)

Values of positivism

'Value-free' science

The values embedded in this approach include the ideal of the disinterested scientist who has no interest in moral or political issues. Accordingly, theories in this paradigm are non-reflexive and blind to their own cultural location.

Prediction and control

The goal of psychology in these applied fields has often been stated as being to 'predict and control'. The idea is that behaviour is reliably predictable based on a set of antecedent factors and if we can successfully predict people's behaviour then it is available for control through manipulation of those causal factors. This positions the scientist as outside the community, as a sort of puppeteer who relies on separate ethical standards to control his or her own behaviour. The ultimate expression of this ethos may be seen in the social marketing approach to health education in which people are overtly manipulated to behave in desired ways using the same powerful tools used by commercial advertisers.

Individual responsibility

Ironically, although the subjects of health promotion are viewed as controllable, they are also individually responsible for choosing the correct behaviour. The use of this approach in health promotion practice has contributed to a moral climate in which individuals are blamed for their poor health. Lupton (1995) has described this dominant ideology of individual responsibility and how it has been used to deflect responsibility for health from the collective (the State) to the individual. Using theories that conceptualize individual responsibility as the sole determinant of health perpetuate this dominance.

Criticisms of social cognitive models

There are many criticisms of the social cognitive models of health related behaviour. Stam (2004) says that these sorts of models are just 'thin' theory, and others claim that they are not really theories, just collections of variables. Leaving these discussions of what constitutes theory aside, it is most useful for us to consider whether these theories provide good explanations of the phenomena or relationships in terms of the criteria that we are interested in. Some critiques along these lines that we might take into account are as follows.

An epistemological fit with the biomedical model of health has been useful for health professionals trying to work together in a medically dominated health care system. Unfortunately, this ready-made alignment has meant that the concepts of health itself are not examined in psychological or social terms. Rather, they tend to be understood as categories of illness and medically defined outcomes. The medical approach to health provides no space for insight into the subjective meaning of health and health related behaviour to individuals, or the dynamic social context of such meanings (Poland, 1992). A more psychological or social perspective would include people's own experience and understandings of health and illness.

The epistemological emphasis on observed variables means no consideration of personal experience, or the fundamental importance of social life. In general there is a total neglect of the social, cultural, environmental and political issues that comprise behaviour. Sometimes factors such as age or gender are included as extrinsic factors to be accounted for, with no explanation of the important socialized and situational meanings of these 'variables' in relation to health and behaviour. In social cognitive models the social influences on thoughts are included as variables such as 'subjective norms'. However, their use as variables that affect individual cognitions does not provide any explanation of the ways in which those individuals are part of a complex social world.

There is a range of conceptual, methodological and predictive problems that have been raised over the years (see Ogden, 2004, for a nice summary, or Conner and Norman, 1998, for some issues from inside the field). Overall, most recent evaluations of the applications of the models in actually influencing behaviour suggest that they simply don't work very well on their own.

Interpreting experience (interpretivism)

For the last three decades there have been increasing calls to go beyond individual cognitions to include the complexity of social life. At the same time there has been an increasing interest and application of interpretivist approaches. Interpretivist theories are concerned with understanding accounts of health from the perspective of the experiencing subject. I will consider two approaches to theorizing from this perspective, phenomenological theories that are concerned with capturing subjective experience, and narrative theories which interpret the ways that we construct and share experiences of health. Because our experience is located in the everyday interactions of social life, such approaches necessarily include the importance of the social world.

Phenomenological approaches

Phenomenological approaches are used with the aim of providing insights into the experience of individuals, 'the lived experience' being the phenomenological tag line that often identifies accounts of research using this approach. A great deal of health related phenomenological research has been directed toward establishing the importance of a person's world and their embodied experience of that world in relation to medicalized practice. In this critical application, medicine is seen as having objectified the patient so that within the regimes of treatment and care, they have become a body of organs and functions amenable to controlled investigation (Radley, 1997). Similarly, social cognitive models are seen as positioning people as a discrete set of cognitions motivated by illness prevention. This objective gaze is seen as dehumanizing, and phenomenologists have set aside notions of the diseased body and the rational mind, to examine people's everyday lifeworld, which include integrated experiences of health and illness. They are concerned to explore insider accounts, body centred meanings and bodily perspectives of the world (Rogers, 2003).

For Husserl, a philosopher of phenomenology, we are beings-in-the-world who cannot be described apart from our world, and whose human world cannot be described apart from us. This is the heart of phenomenological approaches, understanding our intentionality towards the things of our experience. In other words, our consciousness is *about* the world (Crotty, 1998). A focus on embodiment which is particularly applicable to health related research, owes much to the philosophy of Merleau-Ponty who was concerned with our bodies as the source of intentionality and the locus of our being-in-the-world (Radley, 2003).

The lifeworld naturally includes relations with others and these may be understood as an integrated aspect of individual experience of the world. To go beyond individual experience, Schutz (1967) used Husserl's phenomenology as the basis for explorations of social reality. Husserl's injunction was to bracket off, or put aside, our socialized cultural assumptions about the world, so that we may as far as possible have first hand or direct experience of the phenomena, the things themselves. Schutz saw these assumptions as forming part of the essential intersubjectivity of the social world. Our assumptions are shared schemes of meaning with which we make joint interpretations of the things of the world. Using Husserl's prescription for phenomenological bracketing, these taken-for-granted assumptions may be revealed. Schutz was concerned to use this approach to focus on understanding subjectivity in the lifeworld (Scambler, 2002).

Another important aspect of the intersubjectivity of phenomenology is the relationship between the researcher and the researched, and this is highlighted by Radley (2003). In reviewing phenomenological work in health research, Radley concludes that to bracket off taken-for-granted-assumptions involves first recognizing our everyday assumptions about reality. Like Schutz, he suggests that the aim of this bracketing must be to recognize and communicate these assumptions. Thus, phenomenology is not about describing the inner states and subjective experiences of others, but an 'exploration of how we make suffering known to each other' (p. 259).

Narrative approaches

Like the phenomenologists, Bruner (1990) also argues for an approach which recognizes that people's experience and behaviour are shaped by intentional behaviour, and these intentions are the product of culture. Bruner argues for an interactional or cultural model of mind rather than the isolating individual model of Western philosophy: 'When we enter human life, it is as if we walk on stage into a play whose enactment is already in progress – a play whose somewhat open plot determines what parts we may play and toward what denouements we may be heading. Others on stage already have a sense of what the play is about . . .' (p. 34). Furthermore, Bruner suggests that the organizing principle of these cultural meanings, with which we organize our experience, knowledge and interactions in the social world, is narrative.

Many theorists have suggested that human psychology has an essential narrative structure (e.g., Sarbin, 1986; Bruner, 1990). We tend to structure our life story using recognizable and shared narrative forms, we describe the importance of any events in our lives using those forms, and we explain causality and ascribe meaning to events using narrative. A great deal of everyday conversation includes the recounting of stories and narrative construction in this way is a popular way of making sense of the world and self (Murray, 2000). Our ongoing biography is the basis for making sense of ourselves as coherent persons with a past, present and future. For these reasons the study of narrative has proved very useful in exploring people's everyday understandings of health, illness and self.

However, narrative theories themselves are diverse and have been applied in many different ways, and at many different levels of analysis. Some authors have attempted to clarify or organize the use of narrative in the social sciences and Murray (2000) has contributed to these developments by describing four levels of understanding of narrative in health research: personal, interpersonal, positional and ideological. This organization reflects an increasing inclusion of the importance of social structure in the production of accounts and also draws on other theoretical considerations. At the personal level, narrative approaches to understanding people's accounts of their experience are very similar to phenomenological approaches in which the emphasis is on explaining experience and the linking of self with society. At the interpersonal level, the construction of narrative is understood as always a joint enterprise in which at least two persons are involved. This leads to consideration of the social context of the production of the narrative itself and, in research, the role of the interviewer. The positional level includes understandings of the broader social context. This means that the social positions and power relations involved in these co-constructions must be taken into account and this level turns us towards an understanding of the social functions of narratives. The ideological level includes attention to broader social systems of shared beliefs and representations in which narratives are embedded. Murray emphasizes that this schema is not about how narratives are actually structured (they probably include all of these levels all of the time). Rather, it is one way for us to understand the different levels at which different researchers have used the notion of narrative and the notion that the world is mediated to us through stories in many forms.

Interpretivist approaches to people's own experience have contributed a great deal to our understandings of why people continue to engage in risky behaviours, even when they have received and understood the messages about risks to their health, and from the health promoter's perspective it is clearly irrational to continue. For example, why do people, particularly poor people, continue to smoke tobacco when they know the health risks and taxes have made it prohibitively expensive? Many interview studies have now shown that cigarettes have important social and symbolic meanings, such as control over life, security and comfort (e.g., Crossley, 2000a). Similarly, in regard to HIV/AIDS, health promoters wonder why men engage in risky unprotected sex when using a condom seems to be a simple life saving option. Again, interpretative studies have shown that unprotected sex has many more meanings in terms of relationships, resistance and identity (e.g., Crossley, 2000a). Farmer (1994) studied cultural representations of

AIDS in Haiti. He described the way in which the telling of stories about the disease produced shared representations used to explain subsequent experiences of the disease. People do not act as individuals making choices based on a rational consideration of risks to their own health. There are many other more important aspects of social life that influence our intentions and behaviours, which such enquiries reveal.

Values of interpretivism

Humanism

The shift to an interpretivist epistemology includes a change from what Buchanan (2006) has termed the 'scientific model' to a 'humanist model'. The humanist model sees human beings as having free will, and human action as being guided by values and principles. Thus, research is directed towards understanding human values and moral considerations. This shift has been characterized as a reaction to the dehumanizing effect of an individualistic cognitive psychology, which constructed a dehumanizing picture of human being as a mechanism (Parker, 2005) or as 'autistic' (Bruner, 1990).

Reflexivity

The focus on human values rather than mechanisms of cause and effect allows a consideration of the researchers' own values. In turn this opening up of the opportunity for reflexivity lends itself to an analysis of health promotion activity on the basis of values (i.e., Is this right or wrong?) and not in terms of control (see Guttman, 2000). Buchanan (2006) notes the difficulties of this approach: a humanistic model that seeks to include ethical dimensions of agency does not provide the basis for certainty aimed at by the scientific model. He asks, 'When is a reason a *good* reason for a moral judgement?' (p. 2717). And answers that the validity of ethical claims is established by reasoned agreement.

Criticisms of interpretivist approaches

An important criticism is that personal accounts provide very narrow views of experience. Williams (2003) says that although interpretivist research has been illuminating and provided valuable perspectives, there are dangers in privileging lay accounts as *the* valid version of health and social life. The view of the social world from subjective experience is limited to personal interpretations and viewpoints. Williams notes that this is only a partial and potentially misleading view. He uses the example of British interviewees who although poor and in ill health were unaware of the extent of social inequalities in health.

People are not always able to explain their own behaviour. Although interpretivist research has revealed much about people's own intentions regarding their health, and the social and moral basis for many choices, not all behaviour is transparently related to health. Interpretivist researchers ask participants for accounts about their health or health practices. However, many behaviours are an integral part of daily social life, people act in healthy and unhealthy ways according to a whole range of other concerns apart from health (Radley, 1994) and the explanations of these behaviours are not always available to individuals. Thus, interpretive investigations are not always good at explaining health related behaviour because of this gap between people's health related accounts and the structured basis of their everyday practice (Williams, 1995). Researchers using subjective accounts have had to include theories of social or psychological structure from outside the participants' accounts to show how behaviours are enmeshed in daily social life. For example, Chamberlain and O'Neill (1998) used measures of social class to show that differences in accounts about the meanings of smoking and health, understandings of personal control over health, and reasons for smoking are related to the structures of social and cultural life. Crossley (2004) has pointed to the historical nature of behaviours, such as condom use, and described the ways in which these behaviours, are embedded in an unconsciously enacted 'cultural psyche'.

Interpretivist enquiry does not include structural, political or power issues. The humanist values, which inform interpretivist epistemology, locate power in the individual. Studies from this individual perspective are unable to account for power relations beyond individual experience. Thus, these approaches do not grapple with broader societal issues and may result in expectations that individuals or small communities develop power and knowledge. These approaches are not able to incorporate a broader social view and recognition of the operation of social forces that are not always apparent to individuals in their daily lives. Social constructionism, social theories and critical social theories provide a range of approaches that attempt to theoretically account for the operation of that unconscious 'cultural psyche', the everyday social practices that are not about health, and the operations of power differences in our social world.

Alternative realities (social constructionism and poststructuralism)

Social constructionism focuses on the practices of people as part of societies or cultural groups, rather than as autonomous individuals. Language is seen not as a tool to reflect reality, but as the way in which people construct reality together. As members of particular social groups we share discursive resources, or certain ways of talking, which are used in daily life to construct a shared version of reality. Objects in the world, like health and illness and how we should behave, are constructed in language use. Knowledge, attitudes and beliefs are not the property of individuals, but are shared between people through language and multiple circulating texts.

An important aspect of a constructionist epistemology is that recognition of the social construction of knowledge allows for the acceptance of multiple views of reality held at different times or by different cultures. Thus, all claims of knowledge about reality belong to particular times and places. A corollary of this understanding of the constructive role of language is that multiple versions of health may be shared within the same society at the same time. People may draw upon a certain version of health talk according to the social function of their talk. Blaxter (1993) found that middle aged Scottish women gave public and medically authorized responses to survey questions about the causes of illness. The results of a questionnaire survey showed that the women thought that behaviour was the main cause of illness. However, when the same women were given the opportunity in interviews to provide longer accounts of the causes of their illnesses, these accounts were inseparable from explanations of their personal life history couched within a cultural context. As Blaxter's participants showed, questionnaire items may draw on one version of health (the publicly acceptable version of health behaviour) while private conversations draw on more local culturally located explanations for health. The social functions of such talk go further than simply describing experience. They include social interactional 'work', such as defending one's moral standing or legitimating one's behaviour in particular contexts (see Radley and Billig, 1996).

Social constructionism acknowledges the power issues involved in multiple constructions: some versions of knowledge are privileged and some knowledge claims are not socially acceptable. The dominance of biomedical versions of health and illness and the devaluing of 'lay' versions of health is an example of the operation of these discursive regimes in Western society. As an example of the material effects of discursive dominance, the traditional health knowledge and practices of Māori in New Zealand have been repressed through past legislation and ongoing State funding of only Western medical practice. There are several theoretical approaches that may be seen as social constructionist and I will focus briefly on some examples that have been drawn on for health promotion work.

Social constructionist phenomemology

As part of a set of theoretical approaches to underpin health promotion work, Poland (1992) suggested Berger's social constructionist phenomenology as a useful resource. Berger, following Shutz, is concerned with intersubjective systems of meaning, and how culture is constructed and reconstructed through ongoing social exchange. This shared knowledge forms the lifeworlds of individuals and the researcher's task is to identify representations of these shared meanings. The value of this approach is the opportunity to understand culture both as a social structure and as informing individual intentions, experience and identity. Another valuable aspect of Berger's use of phenomenology for health research is that this theory includes the importance of both discursive and embodied life (Yardley, 1997). From this perspective bodies, which are ignored in many social constructionist theories, are included. As individuals we experience the biological (viruses, pollutants), cultural (dietary habits, health care customs) and social factors (working and housing conditions) that influence health as equally real. This relation between biological, social and cultural life includes understandings that we have bodies (to take care of) and also *are* bodies (the 'I' that is the basis of intentional activity).

It is worth noting here that Shutz and Berger's phenomenology, which is firmly based on Husserl's philosophy but is theoretically more social constructionist than experiential, also shows the artificial nature of attempts to categorize theory. Many narrative and phenomenological theorists and researchers would contest being critiqued in the humanist non-critical box, and much narrative research is also undertaken from a constructionist epistemology. It may assist an overview to sort ideas into boxes, but we must beware of taking these boxes too seriously. The important aspect to note here is that theoretical explanations are always available for examination and development.

Discourse theories

Psychology has drawn upon several other disciplines to develop versions of discursive theory for application. Parker (2005) has provided a recent overview of discourse analysis as a way of studying the workings of ideology and power through the constructive nature of language. He outlines four key theoretical ideas that form the basis of these applications: multivoicedness, semiotics, resistance and discourses.

♦ The multivoicedness of language allows us to recognize that variability and contradiction in people's talk (as in Blaxter's respondents) is not error. It is to be expected and is a useful pointer towards the differences in language use and how language works to position people as certain sorts of subjects in social life (e.g., homosexual or gay; patients or clients; prostitutes or sex workers).
♦ Semiotics is the study of how language (including text and visual images) works in these ways to construct certain sorts of people and activities as having particular meanings.
♦ Language is functional. People use language to perform social acts so that language not only describes the world, but it does things. The study of the functional nature of rhetoric in everyday talk shows how people are constantly working to justify, blame and position themselves as certain sorts of people. The study of the functional nature of texts

both historically and in everyday use shows how power relations are per-
petuated in discourses. How some discourses become dominant and how
others are repressed, and how people use language to resist domination.
♦ Discourses may be seen as constellations of certain words and images that
work together to construct objects. Potter and Wetherell (1987) have
developed a theoretical approach to discourse analysis in which they have
termed these chains of images and words 'interpretative repertoires'. In
early work (Wetherell and Potter, 1992), they showed how different repertoires were subtly deployed by speakers in New Zealand to perpetuate
racism. Parker (2005) points to the ideological function of discourses as
presenting versions of reality which control and oppress. 'For example, a
discourse of heterosexuality defines what is deviant, a medical discourse
defines what is sick, and a dominant patriotic discourse defines what is
alien' (p. 90).

The use of discourse theory in health psychology has led to questioning
of the objective reality of biomedical variables, and medical diagnoses, as
well as critiques of whether the biopsychsocial model provides a suitable
framework for understanding health and illness (Yardley, 1997). Discourse
analytic research has been applied in areas such as understanding social
constructions of stress, smoking and sex education (see Willig, 1999).

Poststructural discourse has been very influential in social science enquiries into health. In particular, social scientists have drawn on sociologist
Michel Foucault's (1976) analyses of the operations of power in social life,
including clinical medicine. Foucauldian discourse analysis focuses on the
discursive resources available in a society and points to the ways in which
different versions of reality, and certain subjects and objects are constructed
through language (Willig, 1999). A particular focus has been the ways in
which discursive practices reinforce the power of institutions, such as
medicine, in society (see Morgan, 1999).

Social representations theory

Social representations theory (Moscovici and Duveen, 2000) provides a
broader approach to the functional aspect of the use of language, which
includes both discourse and embodied practice. Moscovici's analysis of the
ways in which psychoanalytic theory was utilized by scientists, politicians
and in popular culture demonstrated how certain words become associated
together and repeated to form particular representations of psychological
life that were shared by members of these groups. Thus, particular words and
images used together to describe an object or idea (such as health) become a
customary part of a culture and are shared by members to interpret and
construct experience. Moscovici explains that the basis of this theory is an
understanding that people communicate 'about objects not as they are
but how they ought to be', which implies the primacy of representations

and systems of shared representations as the basis of knowledge, whether common sense or scientific knowledge (p. 233). Social representations are both shared and produced through social interaction, and combine practical and communicative functions.

Howarth et al. (2004) describe the application of social representations theory to community health research. They note that '. . . social representations theory acknowledges multiple and dynamic knowledge systems about any socially significant object. Differences are seen as consequences of the value and purposes of knowledge systems for different social groups' (p. 232). In addition they make the important point that these different knowledge systems are not theoretically privileged one over the other, or seen as biased, but rather that the representations used by different groups must be examined on their own terms. In general, social representations theory has been used by health researchers to study representations of health across different societies and in different material conditions, the shared representations of various illnesses and what this might mean for sufferers or public health responses, and the manifestations of such representations in practice (see Flick, 2003).

Values of social constructionism

Language

This is the obvious value linking these approaches. Language is now foregrounded as the basis of knowledge and action in the world. To what degree, depends on the theorist. To some, everything reduces to language, others admit to the importance of the 'extra-discursive'.

Relative truth

All knowledge is culturally and historically specific and multiple knowledges can co-exist at one time. This leads to scepticism towards those who claim to have the truth or know the facts.

The social

Social conditions and social relations are prioritized as providing the basis of understandings. Valuing the importance of social interaction in this way takes the emphasis off the individual as representing a problematic case or one whose behaviour needs to change.

Reflexivity

Just as in the interpretivist approach, the ability to critique our own work, question our own values and recognize our own perspective as part of the social interactions of knowledge generation is an important aspect of these approaches.

Criticisms of social constructionist approaches

The apparent relativism of social constructionism has drawn the harshest criticism and the most defensive actions by proponents. The harshest critique of a relativist ontology is that if there is no truth, then all values are equal and any behaviour is admissible. Ultimately, what happens to some of our moral 'truths'? Bruner (1990) takes a pragmatist perspective to choose values of what is good over questions about what is true.

Another issue is the loss of the individual person or the fragmented subject constructed in the multiple discourses of discourse theory. This is a problem for health promotion because although poststructural theorists in particular have demonstrated the illusion of the unitary thinking and behaving person, it is embodied persons who are the object of much health promotion practice. Other theoretical approaches can help fill this gap. For example, narratives provide a sense of a coherent continuous self across time. Willig (1993) proposes the use of critical realism to allow exploration of human subjectivity, or positioning theory to enable exploration of experiences of health (Willig, 2000). Cromby (2007) draws on phenomenology to include embodiment and feelings in discursive analysis. This issue is increasingly being addressed from a variety of perspectives (e.g., see Nightingale and Cromby, 1993).

There are other aspects of these theories that make them difficult to apply in health promotion work. The focus on language excludes much that is important in health and there has been a great deal of discussion over the years in regard to whether a discursive perspective includes the very material aspects that affect health, such as bodies that don't work or lose pieces; lack of money; poor housing; or violence (e.g., Sims-Schouten et al., 2007). Researchers and professionals in health promotion work find that bodies and embodied experiences require more explanation than discourse alone can offer.

Radley (2003) also suggests that discursive approaches take local narratives or discourses of health and move them away from the local context to an examination of broader social forces. In this way they are examined on the terms of the researcher and not the sufferer. A more phenomenological approach preserves the voice of the person who actually experiences health and illness. This is the opposite critique to the one which suggests that interprevist approaches miss out the larger social picture.

Understanding social life (social theories)

The shift in health promotion rhetoric to include the importance of the broader social world on people's health and behaviour also demands a move toward understanding that social world as an entity. A critical approach to research and practice recognizes that the mechanisms constraining people's everyday lives and practices cannot be understood without using social theory (Murray and Poland, 2006). The influence of overarching social structures and mechanisms on behaviour must be taken into account if we wish to make changes at this broader social level to improve people's health. Social theories include cultural models of health that challenge the scientific model and particular aspects of social life that have been described and theorized as related to health beyond direct causal connections. Here I will describe an example of each.

Māori conceptualizations of health

Māori understandings of health are based on a holistic model. According to Durie (1998), Māori see health as a four-sided concept representing four basic beliefs of life: *Te Taha Hinengaro* (psychological health); *Te Taha Wairua* (spiritual health); *Te Taha Tinana* (physical health); and *Te Taha Whanau* (family health). Durie has represented this model of health as *Te Whare Tapa Wha* or the four sided house. As in a house, all sides are equally essential and work together to support well being.

♦ *Wairua*/spirituality is acknowledged to be an essential requirement for health. Without a spiritual awareness an individual may be seen as ill or having lost essential connections and identity.
♦ *Hinengaro*/mental health is understood in terms of thoughts, feelings and behaviour, which are vital to health. Healthy thinking for a Māori person is about relationships. Communication through emotions is important and more meaningful than the exchange of words.
♦ *Tinana*/physical health is the most familiar aspect of health. For Māori the body and things associated with it are part of the sacred world, and are seen in terms of a complex relationship between sacred and ordinary things of the world. In traditional healing practices physical symptoms are seen both in terms of treating symptoms and in terms of restoring the underlying imbalance between the sacred and ordinary and all the parts of health.
♦ *Whanau*/family is the prime support system providing physical, cultural and emotional care. For Māori, *whanau* is about extended relations rather than just the Western nuclear family concept. Maintaining family relationships is an important part of life and caring for young and old is paramount.

Durie's articulation of this model (and the description by others of similar models) has been very helpful for Māori researchers and health promoters who recognize that the Western approach to medicine that had become dominant in New Zealand public health has been detrimental. Durie (1998) suggests that differences between traditional Māori and

Western models of health 'are related as much to time and to balance as to irreconcilable belief systems' (p. 23). For instance, Durie points to recent shifts in Western medicine that take into account the powerful effects of the mind on physical changes, and suggests that there are many similarities between the two systems when one takes a historical perspective of either approach.

Social capital

Social capital is included here as a theoretical construct which has recently become very popular to help explain health inequalities, and to guide community health promotion practice. The social capital concept was developed independently in areas such as sociology, education and political economy. It has been drawn on by public health and development researchers since the 1990s to consider the social effects of inequalities in health. Since its introduction to public health by researchers such as Wilkinson (1999), health researchers have drawn most heavily upon Putnam's (1995) conceptualization of social capital. Putnam has described social capital as a beneficial quality of social life that inheres in the community, not the individual. He defines this quality as 'features of social organisation, such as civic participation, norms of reciprocity, and trust in others', which work together to increase the well being of all. In other words, communities in which people trust one another, care for each other, belong to lots of organizations like church groups or scouts, go on picnics together and enthusiastically contribute to community life by volunteering and voting, will be better off in many ways. However, this use has been criticized as being ill defined, and although this notion has been enthusiastically taken up and measured in relation to the effects of inequalities on population health (e.g., Kawachi et al., 1997), many commentators have been calling for better theories if we are going to use social capital to address inequalities (e.g., Baum, 1999; Campbell and Gillies, 2001; Szreter and Woolcock, 2004; Blakely and Ivory, 2006). Hawe and Shiell (2000) and Macinko and Starfield (2001) have pointed to inconsistencies between the theory and the measures used, and Woolcock (1998) and Portes (1998) noted that the approaches are fragmented. On practical grounds there has been concern that the popularity of the social capital concept allows social policymakers to ignore the material effects of structural inequalities (Muntaner et al., 2001; Fassin, 2003) and to place responsibility for the effects of poverty on the poor (Pearce and Smith, 2003).

Recently, Moore et al. (2006) have suggested that important aspects of the social capital concept have been 'lost in translation' into the discourse of public health. In particular, that understandings of social capital as resources accessed through membership in social networks have been lost. Bourdieu (1986) originally defined social capital as, 'resources linked to possession of a durable network' and seems to provide a theory that includes these important ideas of social networks. Ziersch (2005) and Carpiano (2006) have recently drawn on Bourdieu's theorizing to develop their own conceptualizations and to study social capital and health in neighbourhoods in Australia and the US. However, this use has also been criticized (Stephens, 2008) by noting that Bourdieu's theorizing includes broader understandings of social life beyond just local social networks. It includes understandings of social structure and power struggles that have not been taken into account in these empirical and communitarian applications of his theory.

Values in social theories

Cultural differences

This has not been a comprehensive overview of social theory, however, even these two examples show that a primary value is the recognition of cultural differences in social life and how profoundly they affect our understandings and orientation to aspects of life such as health.

Community

Another basic value in these approaches is people as groups. Not as individuals who belong to groups, but in terms of the very constitutive nature of social life to our being. At this level of analysis, the community is the unit and its values, mores and behaviours are our concern.

Criticisms of social theories

This section on social capital largely amounts to a criticism of the use of a concept that many have noted is ill defined or more of a metaphor than a theory. In addition, as the recent use of Bourdieu's theory has highlighted, such approaches to understanding the broader social aspects of health remain uncritical. That is, they do not include any notions of the political, cultural or historical framework in which inequalities exist.

Durie's model of health has been extremely important and helpful in highlighting and valuing the important differences in health understandings between members of a cultural and ethnic group whose own knowledge and beliefs have been repressed by members of a colonizing culture. However, it does not help us to understand the ongoing activities of repression between these groups in society and their effects on health.

Putnam's work has been drawn upon extensively in public health research to explain various aspects of inequalities in health (Moore et al., 2006). Putnam himself has more recently entered the debates about the pathways through which social capital may affect health (e.g., Putnam, 2004) and his recent work focuses on the benefits of belonging to social groups and networks (Putnam and Feldstein, 2003). However, Putnam's theory of engagement with civic life and socializing through organizations may be seen as essentially a picture of relationships and networks that reflect those of a particular social class, in one particular era. Furthermore, his theory of social collectivity does not account for those who are actively excluded from such groups.

Including power relations (critical social theories)

A critical appraisal of the influence of social structures on behaviour and health includes the recognition that our lives and relationships with others are inexorably shaped by structures of power, but that these are not easily observed. If we wish to begin to understand the relationship between social inequalities and health, then explanations of social stratification and the effects of power relations are essential. However, the broader operations and mechanisms that maintain the situation in which some people have lower status, fewer resources and worse health than others are not readily observable in daily life. We need assistance from social theories that critically address power differentials. Labonte et al. (2005) point to the wealth of social theory available and the complexities of engaging with the multiple versions and competing explanations from well known theorists such as Marx or Weber. To help with explanations of the issues of inequalities in health, sociologists of health and illness (e.g., Scambler, 2002; Williams, 2003) have turned to the works of particular critical theorists such as Bourdieu, Habermas and Freire. Increasing numbers of health promotion researchers have also drawn on these theorists and I will follow their lead.

Pierre Bourdieu

I will begin with Bourdieu because he has already appeared in the discussion of social capital. Pierre Bourdieu's (1977) theory of practice provides a critical look at capital in terms of social competition, as part of a comprehensive theory. In noting that most of our everyday activities may impact on our health but are not *about* health, Williams (1995, 2003) suggested the importance of everyday practice in understanding behaviour from a social perspective. In doing so, he drew on Bourdieu who explains how social structures are unconsciously recreated through 'habitus' or unconscious learned inclination. Accordingly, a great deal of unconscious mastery of the practicalities of daily life informs our everyday behaviour, our social life and our health.

Fine (2001) notes that Bourdieu uses the notion of capital as a metaphor for power. In Bourdieu's theory, 'capital' includes not just economic resources (i.e., wealth) but also the benefits of access to cultural, symbolic and social capital. Competition for access to these interconnected resources is constantly enacted in different fields of practice such as education, sport or commerce, in everyday life (Bourdieu, 1984). Thus capital is a good, but it is not easily available to all. One very important aspect of this competition for resources is the exclusion of members of other groups from access. In *Distinction* Bourdieu (1984) describes the social mechanisms of exclusion through which dominant groups give higher status to certain tastes and objects like art, music, clothing or food and thus maintain their own status symbolically. He has also pointed out that (Bourdieu, 1986), while economic capital is the basis of wealth, social and cultural capital are mechanisms that ensure transmission of capital within wealthy groups. Thus, Bourdieu explains the interrelationship of material, social and cultural capital, and at the same time shifts our health promoting attention from the poor and deprived in society to the role of the wealthy in perpetuating inequalities. Campbell et al. (2004) note the perpetuation of inequalities that is explained by Bourdieu's conceptualization of power: possession of economic, social and cultural capital facilitates the accumulation of more, so that those with the least remain the most powerless.

Jurgen Habermas

Habermas's (1984, 1987, 1990) theorizing of modern social life grew from a tradition of critical enquiry which he situated within a philosophy of language (Crotty, 1998). It is a theory which differentiates between instrumental reason (dominating) and communicative reason (emancipatory). Scambler and Kelleher (2006) have provided a nice summary of the main ideas that frame these contrasts. Habermas distinguishes between the 'system' (economy and state) and the 'lifeworld' (with public and private spheres). He also distinguishes between instrumental action (which is strategic and related to the system) and communicative action (which is oriented to understanding in the lifeworld). Third, he suggests that the state and the economy have been increasingly colonizing the lifeworld through bureaucracy and commodification which limit opportunities for communicative action. For example, medicine has extended its power as an institution, beyond medical consultation to widespread rules about behaviours like diet, exercise and drug use which come to dominate the 'voice of the lifeworld' (p. 224).

This theory has been used in health promotion critique and practice to provide a basis for ethical and participatory practice. Crossley (2001) draws on Habermas to describe how the dominance of instrumental reason in mainstream health psychology produces technical and instrumental outcomes, yet reduces our ability to evaluate the moral worth of our aims. Ramella and De La Cruz (2000) focus on the contrast between communication with instrumental aims and communication for achieving mutual understanding. They suggest that the ideal of communicative action (rather than domination) is an important basis for participatory community health promotion. Similarly, Poland (1992) proposes that critical dialogue as communicative action is a practical avenue for meaningful participation in health promotion practice, rather than the behaviour modification agenda which is based on instrumental action. Scambler and Kelleher (2006) use a Habermasian framework to discuss the importance of new social movements in health (such as environmental protest groups, disability movements or patient groups) as agencies of significant social change which encourage communicative action and lifeworld decolonization. From this perspective such social movements 'are likened by Habermas to new shoots sprouting in the fault lines between system and lifeworld' (p. 222).

Paulo Freire

Crotty (1998) says that no discussion of critical theory would be complete without mention of Freire. At the same time Paulo Freire is probably the critical theorist who has had the most direct influence on health promotion practice. Freire's renown comes from his published work, particularly *Pedagogy of the Oppressed* (1972) and his practice in literacy programmes, work with the poor in Brazil before he was exiled, and subsequent educational work. It is this straddling of critical theory and practice, his emphasis on reflection *and* action, and the expression of explanation as pedagogy, that has made Freiere's work so immediately accessible and useful for health promotion contexts.

Freire's work is in the tradition of Marxist critical theory but also draws on existential phenomenology (Crotty, 1998). At the same time his focus on the constitutive nature of language has links with poststructuralism, and his emphasis on communication as action with the critical theory of Habermas. Ramella and De la Cruz (2000) describe the ways in which Freire's pedagogy informs and develops the Habermasian notion of communicative action for practice. For Freire, the world and knowledge of the world exist in dialogical relationship. Knowledge is not transferred through language, rather knowledge of the world and the words to describe it are the same thing. Knowledge is produced between teacher and student as they communicate. By locating knowledge in 'the intersubjective space created between teacher and student' then the production of that knowledge involves both teacher and student (Ramella and De la Cruz, 2000, p. 277). This approach to knowledge thus highlights the contingent and historically located nature of knowledge.

For the student to understand their own relationship to knowledge in this way is a central aspect of Freire's (1972) pedagogy. He has called this recognition *conscientização* which has been translated as conscientization or critical consciousness (Freire, 1973). Critical consciousness is the development of critical thinking in the student. It contains several stages described by Campbell and Jovchelovitch (2000): 'intransitive thought' when people believe that they have no control over their lives; 'semi-transitive thought' when people try to act to produce change but have fragmented understanding of their situation; and 'critical transitivity' which is the achievement of critical consciousness and a dynamic relationship between thought and action. At this stage people are empowered to change the conditions that are affecting their lives and communicate with others so that whole communities may start working for social change.

Freire's work has been used by health promotion practitioners such as Ramella and De la Cruz (2000), Campbell and Jovchelovitch (2000), and Williams et al. (2003) to contribute to the theoretical basis for participatory health promotion projects that are aimed at empowering communities. The Freirean approach used in these contexts focuses on the development of opportunities and social spaces for participatory dialogue which enables people to problematize everyday life and then develop ways to address the issues raised. 'Freire's concern is to generate the conditions for the partici-pating subjects to pose problems, and to problematise everyday experience by bringing it into communication, understanding and action' (Ramella and De la Cruz, 2000, p. 277).

Values

Social justice

Critical social theories are used by those concerned with social justice, emancipatory values and social change (e.g., Murray et al., 2004). From the perspective of these social theories, the focus of health promotion turns away from changing behaviours toward addressing the relationships between behaviours, and social and material conditions. Practice turns toward participatory community action that enables people to understand and act on the inequitable social structures and on the processes that perpetuate exclusion and marginalization (Murray and Poland, 2006).

Empowerment

Critical theory draws attention to the power differences in health promot-ing practice. It provides explanations for inequalities and observations that privileged groups always capture the benefits of interventions aimed at the disadvantaged (Feachem, 2000). Thus, practice in health promotion based on such understandings values a shift to focus on the systemic or structural dimensions of health issues and the empowerment of those who are systematically excluded.

Moral values

Critical social theorists such as Habermas, encourage a turn towards focus-ing on moral values (rather than on strategic gains that may serve particular interests) as outcomes. This is echoed in Guttman's (2000) concern to shift back from strategic evaluations to values- and ethics-based evaluations of health promotion work. Prilleltensky and Prillelltensky (2003) emphasize that taking power differentials into account is an important aspect of an ethical approach.

Criticisms of critical social theories

One of the enduring issues in social theory is the structure/agency problem. As we move toward understanding the structures of social life, theories lose sight of individual agency and have increasing difficulty in providing us with explanations of how people can change their social conditions. Bourdieu has been criticized on the grounds of determinism; although resisting such claims, he has not developed his explanations of habitus so that we can understand people's ability to change (N. Crossley, 2001). One way to develop this aspect is to consider Bourdieu's own theorizing of communicative action. He has noted that (within a larger sphere of unspoken assumptions and responses) people's willingness to engage in public debate is related to class and habitus. This agrees with and also extends Habermas' own recognition of a general unwillingness to take part in public discussion. Both Bourdieu and Habermas agree that genuine 'public' opinion is formed and fought over in the context of social movements (N. Crossley, 2001). Nick Crossley (2002) has extended an analysis of Bourdieu's theorizing to show how well it explains the important social changing and anticolonizing nature of social movements.

Some social theories are very abstract and difficult to relate to everyday life. N. Crossley (2002) has criticized Habermas for not providing a basis for empirical investigation of his theory. However, a synergy of Habermas's and Freire's notions (and other practitioners have drawn on a range of liberationist theorists to develop practice) has proved useful here.

A danger of Freire's pedagogy is that it may easily be taken as a prescription for practice that *seems* participatory. Frieire's ideas are revolutionary and require some careful meditation to absorb and yet seem to lend themselves to cook book versions. We must be reflexive of our own practice and critical of attempts to set up dialogues that actually have prescribed outcomes and serve other purposes.

When epistemologies clash

In an international context, Barreto (2004) has explained how theories of 'epidemiological transition', or phases of social and economic development that have matched changes in health in the West, do not necessarily apply to developing countries. These theories were developed in the industrialized countries in which the science of epidemiology was also developed. The approach assumes that all countries will follow the steps of modernization that lead to freedom from infectious disease followed by other diseases.

Barreto points to the damaging impact of globalization and neoliberal politics on Latin America and the resulting worsening of health conditions in these countries. The imposition of foreign assumptions about health and technology has not translated into a different set of political circumstances which include foreign domination.

Although there are often several different cultures living in one country the theories and methodologies of health promoters of the dominant culture are likely to unreflexively hold sway as the 'correct' scientific approach to knowledge. Furthermore, dominant Western models of science have been exported along with the globalization of economies to developing countries, while ignoring the local systems and culture. Using critical social theories enables us to recognize cultural and national differences in epistemologies. This recognition of different knowledges and different values is being made by both members of dominant and repressive cultures and by those whose knowledge has been repressed.

Indigenous groups in colonized countries in many parts of the world have made significant advances in recent years in drawing international attention to their struggle for recognition in their own lands and to the impacts of colonization, discrimination and marginalization on health (including genocide, see Durie, 2004). The recognition of differences in theories of knowledge is not always easily resolved. Labonte et al. (2005) describe the challenge for Canadian researchers working with First Nations communities 'where no Western epistemology or rules for quantitative and qualitative research necessarily embody indigenous epistemology, for example, the "truth-telling" of stories' (p. 11). Rather than attempt to resolve questions such as 'whose knowledge claim counts?' these authors have used the principle of an 'ethical space' in which different world views are exchanged until shared agreements about each stage of the research process are reached.

Durie (2004) provides three examples of such practical agreements in health research in Aotearoa to show that Western scientific and indigenous knowledge can be used together. Durie suggests that most indigenous peoples in developed countries live at the interface of Western science and indigenous knowledge, and draw on both in their daily lives. Accordingly, it is useful to work towards drawing these world views closer together. The examples he uses are of research which involved negotiations between the expectations of Māori and non-Māori researchers, and of Māori participants. In a national study of child nutrition, consultation with Māori resulted in several changes to research questions, protocol and analysis of samples of bodily fluids. The results were participation with confidence by Māori and increased confidence and knowledge for both Māori and non-Māori researchers. No attempt was made to fuse the two knowledge systems, rather the integrity of each was included with enhanced results. In a study of the outcomes of Māori mental health interventions, a measure of mental health was developed by Māori researchers using both scientific criteria of robustness and a cultural model of health. This measure was to go beyond clinical measures of symptoms to the holistic interpretation of health important to Māori, and to include measures of mental, physical, family and spiritual health. Although some clinicians were not comfortable with this definition of mental health because it was outside their area of practice, for the most part the measure was accepted by clinicians, consumers and families. The third example is a study of Māori elders in which, to capture a culturally appropriate measure of health, Māori researchers included measures of the quality of participation in certain key areas of Māori society: an index of cultural identity as a measure of health. Again, Durie uses this study as an example of the combination of scientific methods and cultural constructs to successfully develop knowledge from both perspectives.

Assumptions and values of a 'community' approach to theory

Murray et al. (2004) describe the assumptions and values of community health psychology in terms of aims to deepen our understanding of the causes of health and illness in society and develop strategies to reduce human suffering and improve quality of life. They suggest that the values and assumptions of such an approach should reflect the field's underlying moral and epistemological foundations including the recognition of oppression, a concern for social justice, caring and compassion, and respect for diversity. These values underlie the choices of theoretical approaches to the development of health promotion. As part of a discussion of these sorts of issues, von Lengerke (2006) adds that a focus on transdisciplinarity will enable the contribution of broader public health conceptualizations that can account for individual and population influences on health. Murray and Poland (2006) conclude their discussion of health psychology and social action by noting the importance of reflexivity and working to make explicit one's own social location which influences how we understand social relations and frame research questions.

From my own position as a white female New Zealander, I must take account of how this particular social location influences my perspectives and choices. For now, I note that I do have a values oriented position towards understanding the bases of health issues. Observations in epidemiology have been very useful for drawing our attention to the social aspects of health and the effects of inequalities on the health of communities. Thus, I respect the value of such empirical work. However, this work does not provide explanations of causes, and the dominance of applied approaches based in a positivist epistemology has been unhelpful and even damaging to the health of communities. Social cognitive theories are too individually focused and the values of 'predict and control' do not fit with my personal values of democracy and equality. I can remember the first time that I heard this phrase as a student at one of my first health psychology meetings. Qualitative research approaches were being introduced for the first time with an explanation of the epistemological shift that researchers were making in adopting these approaches. The genuinely puzzled response from one traditional health researcher was, 'Well if we want to predict and control, and that's where the rubber meets the road, how will this research help?' This was a shocking response to me, since I was unfamiliar with these aims and naively unprepared for the hostility that met our first forays into socially oriented ways of understanding health. Social cognitive models may help us to focus on how people think about a certain behaviour, like giving up smoking or using medication appropriately, only if the social circumstances are shared by health promoter and client. In the wider social world, messages based on these sorts of theories have worked well for the white middle classes, in other words, those who share the same values as the health promoters and have a privileged position in our society. The point here is that the use of any theory must be reflexive and if our values include concern for broader social issues and social inequalities then we need to shift to more inclusive explanations.

Summary

Theory provides coherently structured explanations for what can be a confusing diversity of observations and insights and points to the ways in which we can conduct research and design interventions to benefit health. In this chapter, I have argued for the importance of theory on both practical and ethical grounds. It is important that we know about the epistemological basis of our understandings of health and are aware of the implications of assumptions about the nature of health that we are using.

Most of the chapter has been taken up with outlines of different epistemological and theoretical approaches to health matters. For the sake of making some sense of differences and similarities, I have structured this account to describe the epistemological background of positivist, interpretivist, social constructionist, social theory and critical social theory accounts. I have also emphasized that there is nothing definitive about this structure. Other researchers and practitioners will not agree with some of the descriptions here. The chief purpose of these accounts is to encourage reflection on the ways in which different theoretical approaches may be applied, the values assumed by different approaches, and the implications of these assumptions for practice. In the next chapter, I will discuss how theories are used to inform different methodologies for research.

Further reading

1 For those interested in following up on social cognitive theories, here are two useful publications from Albert Bandura. The paper gives an account of an important construct in Bandura's theory and cites his foundational work in this area. The 1986 book provides a fuller account of his theory of learning and behaviour:

Bandura, A. (1977) Self-efficacy: toward a unifying theory of behavioral change, *Psychological Review*, 84(2), 191–215.

Bandura, A. (1986) *Social Foundations of Thought and Action: A Social Cognitive Theory*. Englewood Cliffs, NJ: Prentice-Hall.

2 A very accessible, useful and carefully constructed account of the epistemological basis of social research may be found in:

Crotty, M. (1998) *The Foundations of Social Research: Meaning and Perspective in the Research Process*. London: Sage.

3 Two edited collections of papers which grapple with developing discursive theorizing to include subjective experience and embodiment are:

Nightingale, D.J. and Cromby, J. (eds) (1993) *Social Constructionist Psychology: A Critical Analysis of Theory and Practice*. Buckingham: Open University Press.

Yardley, L. (ed.) (1997) *Material Discourses of Health and Illness*. London: Routledge.

Conducting community health research

Introduction

Research questions in health promotion may range from those about the nature of health itself to questions about the ways in which changes that promote health are achieved. If we have a clear account of any health issue and theoretical explanations for its occurrence, what are the appropriate methods to answer such questions? Pearce (2004) advocates the use of methods on the basis of their appropriateness to the issue and the development of new methods as the need arises. He suggests that the broadening international development of public health research has shown how appropriate research methodology differs substantially depending on the public health problem being addressed and the sociopolitical context. Murray and Poland (2006) also advocate flexible methods to suit the aims of the research. They suggest we should choose methods which are based on a clear understanding of the values implied and the theoretical orientation to the health issues in question. It is this theoretical orientation that will determine methodology (e.g., experimental, discourse analysis, action research) and in turn determine the methods (e.g., questionnaire, observation, interview, casestudy). Methodologies inform the use of methods according to theory and epistemology (see Crotty, 1998). For example, a positivist approach to the issue will specify observational and, at best, experimental methods of enquiry, while a social constructionist approach suggests the examination of language and a search for meaning through detailed examination of discourse.

In 1992, following the Ottawa Charter and development of the new health promotion, Poland was recommending the need for a methodological paradigm consistent with conceptual developments in the field. At this time he made a call for methodologies to include the social and policy levels, and to integrate policy, legislative, social, community and individual levels (p. 31). This sounds very comprehensive, but behind such calls was the recognition that health promotion researchers now need a range of appropriate methodologies that include understandings of the very social location of health. The dominance of positivist epistemology and traditional approaches to individual level behaviour change and education has not supported rapid shifts to this broader view of research. However, although the start has been slow, there has been a steady move in the direction of building the use of such methodologies. With an increasingly broader range and diversity of research methods to hand, one of the important aspects of their use is that we choose research methods with a critical view to the implications of their use. This means that we must remain aware of the theoretical and epistemological basis of these methods.

In this chapter, I will describe quite briefly some examples of methodological approaches and how they have been used in health related research. These are examples of use rather than descriptions of particular methodologies and methods that may be found in the many methods texts, both qualitative and quantitative, which are available at present. In structuring these examples, I have not been able to use a tidy one-to-one labelling correspondence between epistemology, theories and methodology. For example, neo-positivist epistemologies provide the assumptions behind a wide range of methods which include both quantitative and qualitative observations. A single well known methodology such as 'grounded theory' (which, although well used in some areas of health research, I have not included below; see Chamberlain, 1999 for a description) has been utilized based on either neo-positivist or social constructionist assumptions. Narrative-based theories and methods are extremely diverse and often may only have the word 'narrative' in common. Thus, the main aim of these examples is to suggest the diversity of research methods available for different purposes in health promotion research, and to provide some direction towards considering the epistemological and theoretical basis of these methods, with their associated assumptions and values.

Observing health behaviours: neo-positivist experiments, surveys, interviews

Research methods based in a neo-positivist epistemology have dominated the social science and health promotion literature, and many readers will be very familiar with this sort of work. The main function of this section will be to touch on aspects of these approaches, note their scope and in particular that both qualitative and quantitative research methods may draw on this epistemology.

Experiments

One of the most influential contributions of social science to health promotion has been social cognitive theories of health behaviour. A great deal of experimental research has been conducted over several decades to test the efficacy of the theory in relation to various health behaviours such as using condoms, eating healthy foods, not smoking and moderate alcohol intake. There are many reviews of this work available now to summarize the successes and shortcomings of the various models. Here I will focus on a few examples of recent work on one small aspect of enquiry to provide the flavour of this approach to research.

One criticism of the application of the theory of planned behaviour (TPB; see Chapter 4) is that it has not addressed the processes by which people's intentions to behave in health promoting ways are translated into action. To test suggestions that a key phase of this process is the formation of an *implementation intention* (a plan to perform the behaviour at a particular time and in a particular place) Jackson et al. (2005) note that studies have shown that participants who form implementation intentions are more likely to eat healthily, take vitamin supplements and attend cervical cancer screening appointments compared to controls. Jackson et al. were interested in the consumption of fruit and vegetables by cardiac patients. Their study randomly assigned 120 participants to a control group, a group who received a TPB questionnaire or a group who received a TPB questionnaire plus implementation intention questions. To measure their daily consumption the participants were telephoned across 28 days to find that they had all increased their daily fruit and vegetable consumption, but that consumption was not improved by implementation intentions. Brandstatter et al. (2001) conducted a series of studies to examine the effects of cognitive load on implementation intentions. In two experimental studies of students, who were given dual tasks, they found that forming implementation intentions enabled initiation of the action, although the effect size was small. Attending to various critiques of TPB, Sheeran and Silverman (2003) tested the model and implementation intentions in a workplace intervention. They embedded an intervention in postal questionnaires completed by 271 participants. Attendance at workplace health courses was doubled for those who had received an implementation intervention compared to those in motivational and control conditions.

Surveys

Similar questions have been examined in this area using survey methodology without controls. Rhodes et al. (2006) used a prospective survey design to evaluate motivation questionnaire items (e.g., exert effort, try hard), intention items (e.g., intend, plan), and implementation intention/ planning items (e.g., specific plans) within the TPB model in the area of physical activity. The results showed that planning did not augment the relationship between motivation and physical activity.

In a different area of health behaviour, a questionnaire was used by Cooke et al. (2007) to predict binge drinking behaviour. Undergraduate students completed a questionnaire containing measures of TPB variables, descriptive norms, anticipated regret and previous binge drinking behaviour, and one week later a measure of current binge drinking behaviour. The results showed that attitudes and anticipated regret predicted intentions, while intentions and previous drinking predicted current drinking. A similar questionnaire was used to test smoking among school children (McMillan et al., 2005). The TPB items (measuring attitude, subjective norm and perceived behavioural control) provided good predictions of both intentions and smoking later. Moral norms and anticipated regret were additionally measured and both explained additional variance in intentions, while only anticipated regret also predicted smoking. Both of these studies were used to suggest that interventions to modify attitudes and induce regret may be effective strategies for reducing binge drinking and smoking among young people.

The TPB has been frequently used to explain precautionary sexual behaviour, particularly in relation to prevention of HIV/AIDS and especially among high risk groups, lately seen as youth and particularly African youth and gay men. Among recent examples of this work, Kok et al. (2007) reported an investigation of the determinants of precautionary intentions among men who have sex with men and who meet sex partners on the Internet. Participants completed an online questionnaire using TPB variables. Attitude, subjective norm and perceived control were good predictors of the men's intentions to use condoms for anal sex with future e-dates. Measures of descriptive norm, personal norm and anticipated regret were also explanatory. Jemmott et al. (2007) used the TPB variables to understand the determinants of HIV risk behaviours, particularly condom use, which are amendable to intervention among Xhosa youth in South Africa. This questionnaire study found that attitude and perceived behavioural control were significantly related to the intention to use condoms, whereas subjective norm was not. These authors concluded that the TPB may be an effective model for condom use and education to emphasize beliefs about the adverse effects of condom use on sexual enjoyment, the ability to negotiate condom use and the ability to use condoms correctly might improve the efficacy of HIV/STD interventions for these young people. In direct relation to education, Hadera et al. (2007) also used a TPB questionnaire to survey undergraduate students in Ethiopia about their curriculum preferences in regard to HIV/AIDS prevention. These authors concluded that the students' motivation to learn was primarily related to subjective norms and was not related to self-efficacy to discuss HIV/AIDS in class.

In general, positivist empirical approaches have proved useful in providing observations of the occurrence of patterns of ill health and the relationships between ill health with material circumstances. Their success in relating cognitions to health and health behaviour is not so clear. A narrow focus on the measurement of thoughts and behaviour has not met the needs of the broader agenda of community health promotion. Williams (2003) notes that neo-positivist methods, such as the epidemiological population survey, decontextualize and atomize information, resulting in the loss of information about the actual dynamics of social relationships (p. 46). We may apply the same critique to all research restricted by methodologies which focus on measurement to the exclusion of meaning. A danger to the success of health promotion comes from the dominance of these approaches in Western social science. For example, knowledge about the causes of illnesses such as HIV/AIDS which is gathered using methodologies that assume individual behavioural causes stemming from cognitions such as attitudes and intentions, and the irrelevance of values has been dominant in Western science. This dominance has been damaging in countries suffering the epidemic (e.g. Campbell, 2003; Mabala, 2006) when it actively excludes knowledge and recognition of the social and structural causes.

Qualitative methods (interviews)

Some qualitiative data is often used in positivist research. For example, interviews are used to gather information for survey questions (a typical approach in developing TPB questionnaires), or to give life to and explain quantitative findings. These methods are largely seen as secondary to the rigorous quantitative approaches. However, there are some uses of qualitative data that have been developed as the focus of knowledge gathering in their own right. For example, researchers in areas such as media studies may use content analysis which involves the methodical counting of instances of particular themes or words. Another qualitative approach that has been developed to extend social cognitive theorizing by using more focused and contextualized qualitative investigations is interpretive phenomenological analysis (IPA).

The developers of IPA (Smith et al., 1999) note that this approach shares with social cognitive theorizing, 'a belief in and concern with the chain of connection between verbal report, cognition and physical state' (p. 219). The methodology is based on the assumptions of cognitive psychology which include an individualist perspective and moves toward the aggregation of commonly reported experiences to provide general understandings of the interplay between cognitions and behaviours. This approach differs from the quantitative methods above in that it includes recognition that the analyst has a role in interpreting the data and constructing the narrative. This move toward the use of qualitative data enables the analyst to include the richer detail of individuals' perspectives, including the importance of their social relationships, on health issues.

IPA is applicable to looking at subjective aspects of health experience, particularly those in relation to identity, the self and sense-making (Smith, 2004). It has been used in health related research to examine topics such as the experience of chronic illness, understandings of the new genetics, sexual and reproductive health practices, or the experiences of health professionals (Smith, 2004). As a particular example, Smith and Osborn (2007) used IPA to study chronic low back pain. Following interviews with six participants they concluded that chronic benign low back pain may have a serious debilitating impact on the sufferer's sense of self which is made worse in relation to others. Their participants' reported that their chronic pain undermined their sense of self and this was sometimes worse than the physical sensations of pain. They worried about a malignant self which affected others and which would be judged by others.

Following social cognitive theorizing, a person's health experiences are understood to be influenced by social life. However, the focus of this perspective is on the perceptions and understandings of the social world by the individual. Giving primacy to individual cognitions does not allow for any broader analysis of the functioning and effects of social values. To make this point, Crossley (2000) uses examples of IPA work with gay men, which reveals the importance of relationships and expressions of love in decisions to use condoms. Although this work reveals the complexities of sexual and social life, Crossley also notes that by stopping at these explanations, this approach is in danger of perpetuating a romanticist image of the self and experience, which does not account for the damaging health effects of particular moral and social structures.

The social perspective: interpretative and discursive methods

Quite a large body of work is now available which examines people's accounts of their illness experience from an interpretive or discursive perspective. Because this work is qualitative and based on linguistic analysis (since the theories assume the primacy of discourse) the notion of qualitative and discursive or interpretative research has become conflated. However, not all qualitative work is based on sound theory. Crossley (2001) has warned against a tendency towards the production of vague unfocused qualitative accounts of health related experiences. Some specific approaches developed from theory are described here.

Narrative

While positivist approaches use qualitative data and the analysis of talk as a way to access underlying cognitions and universal realities, narrative approaches are generally based on the assumption that peoples' own sense of self or subjectivity is constructed in socially available language and narrative forms. Blaxter (1993) demonstrated the importance of this understanding for health research by comparing the results of both a questionnaire survey and narrative interviews with women about their health. She concluded that, although the women understood the health promotion messages about the causes of illness and risks of unhealthy behaviours (and so could check the right boxes on a questionnaire), in the interviews they were more likely to construct their personal sense of health in terms of their individual life story that includes social understandings of self and moral identity.

We use narratives to describe our sense that each of us is a coherent person and that our lives are continuous; thus, narrative approaches have proved particularly useful in understanding subjectivity and the place of illness in our sense of self. Recently, Ville and Khlat (2007) used interviews with people in France about life events to develop these sorts of suggestions. The stories told by their participants supported the notion that building meaning and coherence through narratives (rather than cognitively based constructs such as sense of coherence or meaning) plays a positive role in coping with stressful events and enhancing health. One of the important narrative concepts used in research related to illness itself is the notion of biographical disruption developed by Bury (1982) in relation to the experience of chronic illness sufferers. An illness and the physical and social changes that accompany it are a challenge to a person's identity, and often force a reconfiguring and reinterpretation of life events to make sense of events (Radley, 1994).

Narrative approaches have also been used to examine the relations of illness, self and society. Williams (1984) provided some early and influential analyses of the ways in which sufferers of chronic illness used narrative constructions to make sense of their lives and their selves as participating members of society. For example, he (1993) analysed an interview with a woman with a chronic illness, to demonstrate that sufferers of illness and disabilities develop strategies that depend far more on the moral fabric of society and the individual's place in it, than on coping with specific physical symptoms.

De-Graft Aikins (2004) used the notion of biographical disruption as part of a complex analysis of interviews with sufferers of diabetes and other non-sufferers in Ghana. Both groups identified the disruption caused by the illness to social identity, family and social relationships and economic circumstances. Those with diabetes also talked about the disruption to their body, self and diet. In these sorts of studies concepts from narrative theory are used alongside other methodological approaches to develop integrated understandings of the social location of health.

Discourse analysis

To address the ways in which social life is inextricably bound up with health, some researchers have turned to discourse analysis to examine the social construction of health choices and practices, the ways in which certain constructions may dominate or be resisted, and to critique certain constructions. One powerful aspect of social life that has been examined across time and cultures is morality and our need to be seen as a virtuous member of our society. Discourse analysis methods have been used to show that morality is an important aspect of all health practices. For example, Crossley (2002, 2003) analysed focus group discussions to show that members' talk about health included virtues such as goodness, responsibility and living a good life. The focus group members both employed and resisted these social demands. Such studies form part of a body of work that has examined and critiqued the moral dimensions of recent demands on our health behaviours (to be slim, fit and eat well, and avoid risk of illness) and of our personal responsibilities for being ill. Blaxter and Paterson's (1982) interviews with British mothers and daughters found that women described health and illness as both functional and moral categories. Illness was described as a state of moral malaise and, because health was correspondingly seen as an affirmation of virtuous living, most women wanted to be seen as healthy. Goldstein (2000) and Stephens and Breheny (2007) have more recently shown how women use and actively resist the perceived moralizing of others in making health decisions. This research shows how in everyday life and across social contexts we, as members of any social group, are obliged to present or defend ourselves as virtuous members of our society or to resist blame. Much demonstration of virtue is achieved in talk; when people discuss their behaviour, they reproduce or resist these moral strictures and may also be required to defend their choices to others (Goldstein, 2000; Crossley, 2002; Stephens et al., 2002).

Discourse analytic methods have also been used to show how social constructions of health are shared and shift across time. Lyons (2000) used media representations of menopause in two documentaries to support her arguments that discourses circulated in social life through the media affect people's perceptions of risk and health behaviours, create meaning and influence public responses to certain subgroups of the population, and that representations of health mediate lived experience of physical sensations and subjectivity. In a more comprehensive Foucauldian analysis of shifting discourses used to construct the body, Haraway (1991) compared changes to the way that the body has been conceptualized across the last century with other social and historical changes. Petersen and Lupton (1996) also used poststructural theory to take a critical view of public health activities, including health promotion. This book has provided an influential critique of health promotion from a cultural and sociological perspective. Peterson and Lupton suggest that the focus on psychological, social and physical elements of health is, at its core, a moral issue that deserves scrutiny.

Several other commentators have examined the changing discourses of public health policy (e.g., Robertson, 1998; Porter, 2007). Fullagar (2002) demonstrated the ways in which particular discourses of leisure and healthy lifestyle have been produced through Australian government policy objectives aimed at the body. Sykes et al. (2004) analysed the discourses used in the European Commission's Health Promotion Programme. They identified the use of a 'religious', a 'military' and a 'scientific' discourse to construct the programme and its implementation. They concluded that despite the use of the concept of 'empowerment', the programme as constructed is disempowering through its deployment of hierarchies of power within these discourses. Humpage (2006) has also provided an analysis of the use of policy discourses, in this case the notion of 'social exclusion' which has emerged from European literature. Humpage examines the use of this discourse in the New Zealand context in which there is a tension between the framing of the rights and needs of Māori in terms of cultural experience and the Treaty of Waitangi, and the generic policy concept of exclusion/inclusion. Humpage suggests that it has proved inappropriate to apply a discourse developed overseas to the sociopolitical context of New Zealand.

Although we tend to talk about research informing practice and social policy, it is important to recognize that researchers are also part of the broader social world. Changes in the field of health promotion practice influenced by other social movements may also influence the methodologies used by health researchers. Sato et al. (2004) have described how the workers' health movement in Brazil influenced psychological research and practice in the field of occupational health through everyday multidisciplinary dialogue and action. The workers health movement describes a shift towards a focus on collective health. The involvement of psychologists, whose practice in clinical and occupational areas has traditionally been individually and organizationally focused, has begun to shift towards the problems raised in the field by the workers' movement. For example, social psychologists have become involved in studying discursive practices in relation to work accidents, the social representations of chemical risks, heavy work and the social consciousness of workers with repetitive strain injuries.

Social representations

Social representations theory suggests an approach to discursive analysis that has been used by health researchers since Herzlich's (1973) seminal work in France on the social representations of health and illness. Herzlich identified three types of representations of health used by her interviewees and named them: 'health in a vacuum', 'reserve of health' and 'equilibrium'. Three types of representations of illness followed quite different lines and these were labelled: 'illness as destructive', 'illness as liberator' and 'illness as occupation'. Flick (2000) interviewed German and Portugese respondents to find the same categories of health conceptions with an additional representation of health relating to 'health as lifestyle'.

There have been many studies using social representations to understand conceptions of particular illnesses and to demonstrate competing knowledge systems. Jodelet (1991) used interviews and ethnography to show how representations of mental illness among French villagers influenced the daily exclusionary practices (such as keeping eating utensils separate) of those who hosted recovering psychiatric patients for payment. Howarth et al. (2004) also report work on the representations of mental illness which shows how professional knowledge of mental illness is privileged over the patients' understandings of their illness. These authors also drew on another project to contrast the dominant moral ethos of healthy eating with the experiences and understandings of those positioned as 'at risk' for poor health because of their body size.

Helene Joffe has conducted a programme of investigations into the import of social representations of various illnesses. Joffe and Bettega (2003) interviewed 60 Zambian adolescents (male and female) who live in a population with high risk for contracting HIV/AIDS. Shared representations of the origin, spread and risk of disease linked AIDS to the West, God and teenage girls. Thus, the adolescents believed that while their personal vulnerability was low, the spread of the disease was not in their control but determined by others. Joffe and Lee (2004) examined perceptions of risk in another way by interviewing 50 Chinese women living in Hong Kong about the 2001 avian bird flu epidemic. Environmental factors such as lack of hygiene of Mainland Chinese chicken sellers in Hong Kong represented the causes for these women, which were based on comparisons between old traditions and newer practices. Washer and Joffe (2006) have developed the study of risk perceptions using social representations theory by analysing newspaper coverage of MRSA between 1995 and 2005 to examine the meanings of this disease that circulate in Britain. They found that MRSA is represented as a potentially lethal 'superbug', marking the end of a 'golden age of medicine' in which the discovery of antibiotics has played a key role. The blame for the spread of MRSA is attributed to poor hygiene in hospitals symbolized by the erosion of the 'matron' role, which is associated with lost values of hygiene, order and morality. Thus, Joffe and her colleagues used social representations theory as the basis for 'a detailed examination of how novel threats are assimilated by a society and, in particular, how scientific knowledge is transformed via the mass media into widely held notions that become "common sense" ' (Washer and Joffe, 2006, p. 2148).

The important feature of these investigations into lay representations of health and illness is that, unlike the cognitive models used to explore lay representations of health, illness and risk, social representations theory allows researchers to link their findings to social, cultural and political contexts, which explain the basis and effects of different representations. For example, Flick (2000) related his analysis of the differences in health and illness representations of people living in East or West Germany, and Germany or Portugal, to the differences in social and material living conditions between these areas and countries. Joffe and Bettega (2003) noted that their findings revealed how the representations of higher status groups dominate the social representation of AIDS in Zambia. Teenage girls were seen as the vectors of AIDS in their interactions with 'sugar daddies' and male adolescents. Thus, responsibility was deflected from the powerful men in a capitalist, patriarchal society to blame girls for the AIDS epidemic. Howarth et al. (2004) used studies of mental health patients and women's representations of healthy eating to show how social representations research (like Jodelet's 1991 study) can reveal everyday practices that reinforce exclusion, inequalities and stigma.

Renedo and Jovchelovitch (2007) have developed the social representations approach to understanding expert knowledge and its relationship to health. In their study of professionals working with homeless people in London, they point to the impact of health professional knowledge on health and care policies for the homeless. However, the health professionals work between the definitions of the statutory sector, which limit homelessness, to intentionality and 'lack of a roof over one's head', and the voluntary sector whose understandings take into account the whole person and the heterogeneity of the homeless population and their complex and differing needs. The interviews with professionals showed that their representations of homelessness include the definitional clashes, dilemmas and contradictions of this situation. The representations of the health professionals showed that homeless people could be seen in both ways and these contradictory representations (theorized in social representations theory as cognitive polyphasia) suggest the importance and the complexity of health promotion work.

Howarth et al. (2004) suggest that such social representation research is potentially useful to health promotion but should move towards a more participatory approach. Krause (2003) has provided an example of how this might work. Krause describes a participant action research process in which a self-help group whose members suffered from inflammatory bowel disease, worked towards transforming social representations of the disease. Beginning with Herzlich's work which showed that social representations of illness affect the way people cope with disease, and the recognition of the validity of different representations, Krause suggests the possibilities for change. In her example, a self-help group in Chile worked to change their own shared representations from those of their disease as a serious handicap to 'normalization' with more restricted attention to the illness. These representational changes also resulted in changes in relationships with health professionals and with society in general.

Observing in social context: ethnography

Ethnography is the tool of anthropologists and medical anthropology although used by researchers from other disciplines. This qualitative approach has much in common with the discursive approaches described above in terms of methods (such as interviews and observations) and the theoretical bases which lead to an emphasis on understanding the social location of health using fine-grained analyses of experience. Furthermore, ethnography has a commitment to thick descriptions of phenomena that are contextualized within holistic views of social life. Chapman and Berggren (2005) describe these methods as '. . . the culmination of listening, observing and experiencing so many stories that they start to overlap, change and repeat until the spectrum of responses has been collected and some agreement on general themes and patterns is established' (p. 151). Cook (2005) suggests that critical ethnography is an appropriate approach to exploring issues in health promotion. These issues, such as the determinants of health including income, child development, education, social support and work conditions, which are influenced by class and gender relations, local and global economies, and cultural norms, are difficult to take into account using the dominant methodologies in health research.

Nguyen and Peschard (2003) provide a comprehensive review to support their argument that ethnography is a useful way to develop our knowledge of the basis of inequalities in health. Pointing to the inadequacies of existing methodologies, like Cook, they propose that ethnographic approaches are able to take account of complex multifactorial mechanisms. They further provide a theoretical framework for research projects that understand affliction as the embodiment of social hierarchy and use ethnographies to examine the ways that inequalities are embodied; how therapeutic power is legitimated; and how groups respond to misfortune. These authors provide detailed examples of work addressing these issues. Similarly, Chapman and Berggren (2005) specifically consider racial and ethnic disparities in health and describe how ethnography may be used to provide new knowledge about inequalities. For example, ethnographies have been used to document internal colonization and the lives of the disadvantaged. In addition, ethnographers have documented the interactions of disenfranchised peoples with those in power, the operation of White privilege in many settings, and re-examined from the participants' perspectives, the 'risk' behaviours of particular groups in the context of the economies and social negotiations that inform them.

Ethnographic work engages with people's lives to contribute to broader social critique. Scheder (cited by Chapman and Berggren 2005) studied diabetes in migrant workers to reveal economic and racialized stress and to critique the social, political and immigration policies that limit the individual's ability to cope. In a related area, Edmondson (2003) used ethnographic evidence to demonstrate the complex and culturally diverse nature of social capital. Her study was designed to contribute evidence to the moral and political debate about social capital and health in public policy.

One of the best known ethnographers in health research is Paul Farmer whose long-term ethnographic study of AIDS has been influential in developing understandings of lay representations of health. Farmer (e.g., 1994) documented the elaboration of a detailed and widely shared cultural model of AIDS in Haiti and used ethnographic processes to reveal structures of meaning in which people's understandings were embedded. Of this process he has said:

> Understanding the processes by which a new illness representation came into being required a constant shuttling back and forth between individual and collective experience, between 'macro' and 'micro,' between shifting narrative structures and enduring frameworks that, while subject to change, nonetheless serve as a grid helping to frame illness experience. In a previous study of another illness in rural Haiti, 'the need to connect personal illness meanings with larger political and social systems' was underlined
>
> (1994, p. 801)

Farmer's (1999) work has informed understandings of inequalities by demonstrating that the HIV epidemic 'tracks along social fault lines' and affects those whom poverty and social exclusion makes vulnerable (Nguyen and Peschard, 2003). Castro and Farmer (2003) have provided detailed case studies of individuals' experiences of HIV/AIDS and tuberculosis in Haiti. These authors describe how the social situation including racism, sexism, political violence and poverty are rooted in historical and economic processes. These forces which they name 'structural violence' are an integral part of the stories of vulnerability to these preventable diseases.

Shared methodologies

It may already be apparent that there are some fuzzy boundaries between these methods as used by health researchers; there are many overlapping features of the different approaches whatever we call them. Once you read any of the research reports in more detail it will become clear that many researchers are drawing flexibly and creatively on the approaches available when it comes to actually conducting investigations. For example, Farmer, whose work I have described above as ethnographic, uses peoples' narratives about illnesses and their own broader experiences as an important aspect of his work. In his paper (Farmer, 1994) about the use of narrative, he says that one approach to tracking the development of understandings of AIDS from its introduction to its manifestation as an epidemic is '. . . simply by attending more closely to the way in which illness (and other misfortune) is worked into narrative renderings of broader experience' (p. 801).

This approach reminds us that just because we name and describe methodologies and methods they are not necessarily exclusive. Researchers may draw on a variety of methods as long as they share the same epistemological assumptions. Murray (2000) uses examples that show how the use of concepts from discursive theory and rhetorical analysis reveal the social and interpersonal positioning work that is achieved in narratives. Harré and Gillet (1994) have explained how this combination works with their theoretical notion of the 'positioning triad' in which all three elements are seen to be an integral part of every discursive act: an evolving narrative or story line, the speaker's rights, duties and obligations within the local moral order, and the force of the social act that is performed by the speaker. This has proved to be a useful analytic schema for understanding discourses about health decisions which turn out to be made quite differently in the broader social world than a medical decision making scheme would suggest (Stephens et al., 2004)

In a different sort of combination, Murray et al. (2003) used both social representations and narrative theory to explore the socially shared representations of personal responsibility and lifestyle in the everyday beliefs about health and illness held by baby-boomers in Canada. Murray (2000) points to the importance of social representation theory in analysing narratives at the ideological level: the level at which society's systems of beliefs are developed, shared and represented in narratives. De-Graft Aikins (2004) has used narrative theory and social representations to show how people use both lay and medical concepts together flexibly in ways that accord with medical goals. Her findings challenge the traditional ways of understanding lay beliefs, which always contrast traditional beliefs with biomedical systems. However, she is also able to point to how the focus on beliefs and practices ignores the practical and structural barriers to self-care which were particularly salient for diabetes patients in Ghana.

One methodology that invites the inclusion of other approaches is participatory action research (PAR). In turning to a discussion of its use we also turn from methods in which the researcher is using their expertise to answer questions about the lives of their participants, to approaches that focus on the role of the subject of health promotion practice. Participants take an active role in answering their own questions about health.

Researching and doing – participatory action research

PAR combines knowledge development with action and change, and involves those for whom the change is designed in the research process. Thus, PAR is quite different from conventional health research because the knowledge is directly related to action and change for improvement, rather than to understanding (Patten et al., 2006). In this way PAR is both a research methodology and a model for health promotion practice (which is the topic of the next chapter in this book). It sits across both topics and is another example of the difficulties of categorizing. It is included in this chapter because PAR is an important research methodology for health promotion owing to its direct applicability to the business of health promoters.

As a research method, PAR has many different proponents, but most draw upon Kurt Lewin's field theory and his work which introduced the term 'action research' (e.g., Lewin, 1946). Most also agree on two central features: first, action research is based on what is presently happening in the field, and this leads to the cyclic nature of the research. Within any action research cycle there are phases of planning, acting, observation and reflection, leading to re-planning. Second, the research is conducted by and for all stake holders. In this way PAR rejects the traditional model of the expert researcher, and sees any research project as a collaboration between different stakeholders (e.g., researchers and those whose lives may be changed) with reciprocal exchange of knowledge and equal valuing of all understandings. New knowledge is understood to be only based in social relations and action.

Examples of PAR

Kemmis and McTaggart (2000) have developed a popular model of PAR that is well used by researchers in the field. Their model addresses 'community, organizational, ideological and power-related issues in a social situation' (Waterman et al., 2007). They describe the four phases of the research cycle as: planning (examination of the problem and forming practical objectives); action and evaluation; reconsideration of the plan in the light of the new data; and revising the plan. Bradley et al. (2004) describe three cycles of such an action research project designed to increase the capacity (seen as collective efficacy) of young people at risk in Australia. Drawing on observations and interviews to establish the issue, and critical theory and associated techniques to provide a forum for participation, the researchers moved through three cycles of the research. They arranged for a 'public conversation' about youth at risk, set up a youth theatre group (Voices) who were enabled to address their problems, and facilitated participants in this group to influence the local council's support for a full-time youth worker. Across these cycles, the first was seen as not successful, although its evaluation did shift the researchers towards the more successful strategy of directly involving young people themselves.

Just as Bradley et al.'s research goals were based on the community oriented concept of capacity building, so other researchers have used PAR to work towards similar goals such as empowerment. Williams et al. (2003) aimed to increase the role of members of marginalized groups in policy advocacy for changes in the determinants of their well being. These researchers used a narrative approach based on Freiere's critical pedagogy. The participants, an advocacy group of eight women of mixed ethnicity from a deprived suburban area in New Zealand, and the facilitator told stories relating to particular issues. The stories affirmed the importance of culture and identity to the women and developed into stories of injustice, both political and personal, in relation to housing conditions. A feature of PAR noted by these researchers is its capacity to produce surprising results.

In this case they note that nobody 'anticipated the extent to which the political, cultural and gender identities became inseparable from those of policy advocacy, and essential to any social action outcome that might be considered "empowering" ' (p. 35).

A powerful use of PAR has been described by Brinton Lykes (e.g., 2000). Lykes has drawn on the liberation psychology of Martín Baró (based in turn on Freire and others) to work with women in Guatemala who have suffered the ongoing effects of war and human rights violations. This theoretical basis includes the importance of the co-construction of meanings and the principles of working *with* people – those of PAR. Thus Lykes, who has been working since 1986 with rural health promoters, adopted this approach to develop participatory workshops with a growing group of women. From this work a PAR project was developed using oral history interviews and photography to communicate, analyse and share the women's stories. The women photographed their own life stories and the stories of others, taking their tools to neighbouring villages and eventually creating an exhibition, travelling with it around Guatemala. These stories of daily living told of war and its ongoing effects including poverty. The women also developed sensitivity to the many forms of violence and recovery strategies in their region (Lykes et al., 2003). Within the groups the women developed ethical strategies for using these tools, and strategies over time for analysing and presenting their collective record to others, and critically reflecting on their own and the group's work – 'developing a shared vision towards collective action for change' (Lykes, 2000, p. 393). An important aspect of this work emphasized by Lykes is the ongoing reflexivity of the PAR approach. First, this reflexivity involves the recognition of power relations and the complexity of negotiating selves in transnational work. Those from privileged situations must work to resist the advantages of privilege, while using that very privilege to contribute to the health of communities. Second, Lykes notes that one must be constantly engaged in acting, reflecting and critiquing, then acting on the basis of that critique. The role of the facilitator in the relationships that allow these activities is crucial and yet the most important aspect is to be able to work and think *with* the people for whom we seek 'greater economic justice and social equality'.

Photovoice

Photovoice is one of the chief methods used by Lykes in the PAR project mentioned above, and it deserves some attention here because photovoice (along with narrative and other discursive approaches) is a method that is particularly appropriate to PAR methodologies; because it provides a means of expression beyond words that is more appealing to many groups; and because it is becoming increasingly popular with community health researchers. For Lykes (2000) photovoice, as described by its originators (e.g., Wang et al., 1998), was an important resource that fit the PAR methodology as articulated by the group. Using photographs enabled the women to document their experience of violence and its effects through images they chose and created, and to situate these images in the context of their 'cultural, religious, labor, and community practices that had been deeply threatened by the war' (p. 391). The process has had multiple outcomes as the women shared, worked together and developed a focus for changes in their lives.

Photovoice has been used in several local health promotion projects in different countries and situations worldwide. It has proved to be useful in working with young people in Western countries who are familiar with the technology and find pictures more immediately engaging than other methods of communication. In a typical example of this sort of use, Wilson et al. (2007) describe a youth empowerment intervention in the US that aimed to provide underserved early adolescents with opportunities for civic engagement around issues of shared concern. The project was facilitated by young people (older students) who were guided by a curriculum that was adapted after evaluation of the first cycle. The participants met in after-school groups to learn about photography; use cameras to photograph the good and bad things in their environment; develop critical analysis by discussing and writing about their photographs; and develop social action projects that were initiated by each group. One difficulty noted by the researchers was the problems experienced by these young people in shifting to understandings of wider causes of local problems and moving from critical discourse to social action. The development of the approaches to these aims is part of the ongoing reflection of the team and is the opportunity for reflection on these aims and those of the young people involved.

PAR and other methodologies

Although based firmly on complex theories of knowledge generation, PAR has also been developed as a model for research and practice that can draw on a range of different methodologies. As we have seen in the examples above, narrative approaches or community arts such as drama and photography are natural methods for use in participatory projects – these are methods that use cultural values and skills already well honed or quickly understood by any new researcher. In addition, more abstract theories are applied within PAR projects. Bradley et al. (2004) and Lykes (2000) have based their choices of PAR methodology on understandings from critical social, dialogical and liberation psychology theorizing. Krause's (2003) PAR project with a self-help group described above used a methodology based on social representations theory. Cook (2005) describes the use of critical ethnography in participatory approaches by using an example of research that explored nutrition inequalities and then engaged participants in exploring the social roots of their problems and choosing appropriate courses of action (in a similar way to the intervention of Wilson et al., 2007, above).

However, Cook (2005) also sounds an important note of warning about this type of combination of methodology. Although PAR and critical ethnography share the aims of changing existing social structures, they do not share all methodological assumptions. She notes that although ethnographical research participants may have a voice and can challenge the researcher's emerging analysis (if given the opportunity), they do not have the control over the research process that they might have in a truly participatory process. 'In purely critical ethnography projects, the research questions and the form of data collection remain the domain of the researcher, following traditional researcher and participant roles' (p. 134). This does not mean that critical ethnographers cannot adapt their methodology, but it does point to some powerful assumptions and methods that do not shift readily into a participatory approach. While it is appealing to be conducting participatory research, this may not always be appropriate to the aims of the project. It brings us back to the importance of reflexivity and awareness on the part of the researcher of their aims and assumptions. A participatory approach must be grounded in an appropriate set of assumptions, and not be used as a friendly label that masks other intentions. Researchers must acknowledge these differences as they arise, and watch out for instances when they are slipped over or hidden behind appealing labels. Some more specific examples of aspects of these sorts of models will be seen in Chapters 6 and 7 and will provide you with some opportunity to evaluate and compare the different uses of this sort of approach.

Why focus on methodology?

It is important that health researchers maintain an awareness of the range of different approaches to research in health that are available and their theoretical and epistemological bases. In devoting a chapter to brief examples of these methodologies I hope that we can maintain a balance between two dangers for the researcher. The first is a slavish devotion to the methods and rules of a particular approach to the point that we lose sight of the understandings behind the methods or opportunities to use research methods creatively. The second, is that if we get too unconstrained and are not creative enough, we may lose sight of any methodological justification altogether and produce research that is not very informative and a waste of participants' time and goodwill.

In regard to the first issue, there have been some critics of a slavish focus on methodology in health research in both quantitative and qualitative approaches. Chamberlain (2000) has summarized commentaries in regard to psychological research and pointed to several tendencies of researchers and reviewers in qualitative research in particular, who have succumbed to 'methodolatry' such as: an emphasis on locating the proper methods and the proper steps; a focus on description rather than interpretation; and looking for prescriptions to avoid theory. Certainly one of the chief dangers in focusing on methods is that the theoretical understandings get lost and meaningless data is produced.

On the other hand, there is a danger that, as we cast aside the strict boundaries that were developed within positivist approaches to science, there is no wisdom to guide our next steps. We are not all natural theorists and creative researchers. Nick Crossley (2002) a medical sociologist, has pointed to one serious danger of a shift into unguided areas beyond theory. In rejecting positivist frameworks without such guidance we may be left with 'eclecticism and empiricism (i.e., the bundling together of interesting empirical observations)' (p. 16). In general, the reader does need to be alert to the dangers of such atheoretical research. The authors of many papers may claim to be using phenomenology or narrative theory or discourse analysis. In actuality, many are using empirical observation whose results are discussed in ways that reveal all the values of positivism, without its accompanying methodological strengths designed to address reliability and validity.

In the end, these dangers are not two opposing issues but revolve around one central set of issues: the need to have sound theory that is the basis of the research question, the methods, the analysis and application of findings, and the need to be reflexive about these issues. We may be guided by other theorists and researchers who develop new and insightful ways to understand the world, but we must be able to be ongoingly critical of our own use of these methods.

Summary

This chapter complements the previous theory chapter by focusing on the methodologies that develop from different theoretical approaches. The examples of different methodologies described here have been drawn from those used in the health field. The examples of experimental, survey, discursive, ethnographic and participatory approaches show that the same data collecting methods, such as surveys, observations or interviews, may be used from quite different epistemological perspectives. Accordingly, although we do not want methodologies to become fixed and rule bound, it is important to be aware of the methodological basis of research. The same principle applies to the use of theory to develop interventions in health promotion practice. In the next chapter, I will review some examples of the application of theory and research to develop models for interventions.

Further reading

1 An edited collection with an emphasis on the theoretical bases of research and practice, focusing on social cognitive approaches to health behaviour:
Glanz, K., Rimer, B.K. and Lewis, F.M. (eds) (2002) *Health Behaviour and Health Education: Theory, Research, and Practice*, 3rd edn. San Francisco, CA: Jossey-Bass.
2 An edited collection introducing a range of qualitative approaches for use in health psychology:
Murray, M. and Chamberlain, K. (eds) (1999) *Qualitative Health Psychology: Theories and Methods*. London: Sage.
3 An edited text which draws on research experience to describe qualitative and quantitative methods employed in health research. It covers issues such as research ethics, comparative research, the use of mixed methods and the dissemination of research:
Saks, M. and Allsop, J. (2007) *Researching Health: Qualitative, Quantitative, and Mixed Methods*. Thousand Oaks, CA: Sage.
4 An edited collection covering a range of very interesting issues in participatory research methods:
Minkler, M. and Wallerstein, N. (eds) (2003) *Community-based Participatory Research for Health*. San Francisco, CA: Jossey-Bass.
5 An edited collection which is focused on the health related applications of discursive research:
Willig, C. (ed.) (1999) *Applied Discourse Analysis: Social and Psychological Interventions*. Buckingham: Open University Press.
6 A text that provides an overview of participatory action research, its strands, underlying tenets and practice using examples:
McIntyre, A. (2007) *Participatory Action Research*. Thousand Oaks, CA: Sage.

Theories and models for community health promotion

Introduction

This chapter overviews theoretical approaches to health promotion interventions. Descriptions of the theoretical models that are being used in many parts of the world at present will be illustrated with references to examples from work in several different countries. This will be followed by a discussion of the values that underly the choices of theoretical models and the ethical issues involved in making these choices.

The models described in this chapter draw on the social theory and research used to understand health outlined in preceding chapters, and on additional theoretical accounts of change. In practice, health promotion interventions need to draw on different theories for different parts of the work. For example, theories of health may explain the various influences on health which are then seen as the targets for an intervention. However, these theories do not necessarily explain the ways that we may address or change those influences. Thus, a health promotion worker may need to draw upon additional theories such as those regarding education, communication or social movements to help implement desired changes.

For applied purposes, theory is used to develop models of health, behaviour and social relations that include change. Some models draw on several theoretical bases and empirical evidence to describe the factors that influence health. Glanz et al. (2002) describe the importance of theory in health behaviour change and suggest that '*Models* draw on a number of theories to help understand a specific problem in a particular setting or context. They are often informed by more than one theory as well as by empirical findings' (p. 27). Here, I use the word 'model' to refer to the use of any coherent plan for action by health promoters that is based on more or less explicitly acknowledged theories.

Models for community health promotion practice

Just as there are many different ways of understanding community, there are different conceptions of community intervention. For example, community-based interventions may take a population approach in which the focus is on the social context and the behaviour of all community members. Or a community-based intervention may target only those members of a particular community who are seen as being at risk of poor health outcomes. Some models are based on conceptions of the person as an individual affected by aspects of a wider system, and others take the theoretical perspective of the person who is an intextricable part of their social world. To describe health promotion models that take a broader view of health, and to examine some of the different approaches to models for intervention, the following account is structured in terms of 'ecological' models, 'social determinants' models, and 'local and cultural' models. These are loosely descriptive labels only, which have been used to structure the diverse range of models that are available for different purposes. In addition, I examine health promotion messages and the media and different ways in which the broader structural and political issues in health have been addressed. Within each category models are described in terms of their theoretical basis, with some examples of their application and some critiques and problems that have been encountered using each approach. To close this chapter I discuss different ways of assessing the values and ethical issues involved in choosing models of health promotion practice.

Ecological models

Social ecology

An increasing focus on community as the basis for health promotion has developed from the recognition that people's behaviour is influenced by their environment. Social ecology has played a very important role in the development of broader community-based models for health promotion. 'Ecology' is a term that describes the interrelations between organisms and their environments, and as a basis for research has moved from its origins in biology to provide disciplines such as psychology, sociology and public health with models for understanding people's relations with their physical and social environment. In 1992, Stokols outlined the importance of a social ecology of health promotion in the *American Psychologist*. He described the ways in which social ecology has developed to focus on the social, institutional and cultural contexts of people–environment relations as well as on the geographic environment of human ecology. Stokols' account (1992, p. 7) describes four core assumptions of a social ecological perspective on health promotion:

♦ The healthfulness of a situation and health of its people are influenced by multiple and interacting facets of the physical (e.g., geography, architecture, technology) and the social (e.g., culture, economics, politics) environment.

♦ Human environments are highly variegated in terms of physical and social components, and the meanings or interpretations of these components from a multitude of perspectives. This has important implications for health promotion.

♦ Participants in environments may be described at varying levels from individuals, groups, organizations, larger aggregates, to populations. A social-ecological approach should incorporate multiple levels of analysis and diverse methodologies.

♦ The social-ecological perspective incorporates concepts from systems theory such as interdependence, homeostasis and negative feedback to understand dynamic interactions between people and their environments. Systems theory suggests a complex of mutual influences in which physical and social features may influence the individuals' health, but the participants in those settings are also influencing the healthfulness of the environment. The levels of environments, from individual to population, are seen as complex systems so that the immediate groups are also part of broader more complex organizations.

In general, social ecological approaches have included interactions between the developmental and psychological characteristics of the individual (e.g., norms, values, attitudes), their interpersonal relationships (e.g., family, social networks), neighbourhoods, organizations, communities, public policy, the physical environment and culture. In these models individual behaviours are understood to be the result of these interactions and, accordingly, changing health behaviours and health outcomes requires addressing these social and environmental influences. Such

> interventions may include family support (as in diet and physical-activity interventions), social network influences (used in tobacco, physical activity, access-to-health-care, and sexual-activity interventions), neighborhood characteristics (as in HIV and violence-prevention programs), organizational policies and practices (used in tobacco, physical-activity, and screening programs), community factors (observed in physical-activity, diet, access-to-health-services, and violence programs), public policy (as in tobacco, alcohol, and access-to-health-care programs), the physical environment (used in the prevention-of unintentional-injuries and environmental-safety programs), and culture (observed in some counteradvertising interventions).
>
> (McLeroy et al., 2003, p. 531)

Stokols (1992) also suggests that the social-ecological perspective must use interdisciplinary approaches to health promotion. Because of the complexity of the different aspects interacting to affect human health and the healthfulness of any environment, knowledge from medicine, public health, and the behavioural and social sciences must be combined.

Bronfenbrenner's ecological model

Bronfenbrenner's (1979) ecological model has been particularly influential in encouraging multidisciplinary work. Initially developed as an approach to human development, the model has had widespread influence on the way social scientists approach the study of human beings and their environments, and has been credited with breaking down barriers between the separate disciplines in the social sciences. It has been drawn upon widely by community psychologists and used as a basis for understanding health promotion issues (e.g., Cornish, 2004). Bronfenbrenner's model describes four levels of nested systems which are increasingly distant from the person. He called these the *microsystem* (immediate environments such as the family or classroom); the *mesosytem* (connections between immediate environments such as home and school); the *exosystem* (external environments which indirectly affect development, e.g., parents' workplace); and the *macrosystem* (the larger sociocultural context). Each system contains roles, norms and rules that can powerfully affect individuals. An important aspect of this model is that because it is essentially a developmental model, each level is understood in terms of the individual and the way in which the broader systems enter the individual's experience.

Social ecological models in practice: the physical environment

Although practitioners do not always explicitly call upon particular theories or models of interconnected environments, the social ecological approach has been very influential in shaping health promotion practice. An ecological approach is often referred to in justifying the importance of including the environment. For example, ecological models have been referred to as justification for exploring the importance of the physical environment for health issues. In particular, exercise and its negative relationship to several health outcomes, such as to obesity, CHD and diabetes, has led to an interest in the physical environment as an important influence on people's ability to actually engage in exercise. Practitioners realize that even if people understand the issues and are motivated to increase their exercise, the physical environment may be a significant limitation. Saelens et al. (2003) have argued for the use of ecological models which suggest that a combination of psychosocial and environmental variables will best explain the influences on physical activity in communities. They reviewed the evidence for the important variables to suggest a model of predictors of walking and cycling behaviour that includes the effects of three important aspects:

- *Neighbourhood environment*: e.g., density, connectivity, land use, safety, walking and cycling trails, parks, neighbourhood topography and aesthetics.
- *Individual factors*: e.g., age, gender, income and car ownership.
- *Psychosocial factors*: e.g., self-efficacy, perceived benefits, perceived barriers, social support and enjoyment.

Walking alone has been identified as the most common physical activity and the activity people are most amenable to incorporate. Owen et al. (2004) have provided a review of encouraging, although mixed, support for the environmental influences that may increase people's tendency to increase walking. Among the factors that they identified as associated with walking were: the aesthetical attributes of the neighbourhood; the convenience of facilities for walking (such as sidewalks and trails); the accessibility of destinations (like stores, parks or beaches); and people's perceptions about traffic and busy roads. The attributes associated with walking for exercise were found to be different from those associated with walking to get to places.

Wendel-Vos et al. (2007) systematically reviewed the evidence for the determinants of a broader range of physical activity including neighbourhood walking, bicycling, vigorous sports, active commuting, general leisure time physical activity, sedentary lifestyle, moderate physical activity, and a combination of moderately intense and vigorous activity. Among their results, social support and having an exercise companion were found to be convincingly associated with all the different types of physical activity. Availability of physical activity equipment was convincingly associated with vigorous physical activity, and sports and connectivity of trails with active commuting. Other possible, but less consistent, correlates of physical activity were the availability, accessibility and convenience of recreational facilities. Overall, these authors concluded that of all the expected environmental determinants, supportive evidence was found for very few.

The ecological models suggest the importance of including broader influences of environmental factors on people's behaviours, and there is some evidence to support this. However, such models do not include good explanations of exactly how the environment, or the broader macro levels of a person's micro system, actually affect their everyday behaviour. Owen et al. (2004) suggested the need for better theorizing in this specific area of influences on exercise behaviour. They have proposed the use of theories that include consideration of habitual individual behaviour which is shaped by the physical environment.

Social ecological models in practice: the social environment

When the social environment is taken into account, the behaviour of individuals is understood as being the result of not just their knowledge, values

and attitudes, but as the result of many social influences including interpersonal relationships, organizations and communities (McLeroy et al.,
2003). Thompson and Kinne (1999) have described a social change model
based on systems theory. Their proposed model is a synthesis of theories of
social change at the different levels of individual, organizational and community change. They draw on appropriate theories to explain change at
each level of their model which include:

♦ *Individual level change*: Here there are many theories available in the health
  promotion literature, including the health belief model, theory of
  reasoned action and social learning theory.
♦ *Organizational level change*: There are many theories of change in the
  organizational field. These take account of organizations as systems and
  communities in their own right, and explain collective action, social
  movements and organizational development in these contexts.
♦ *Community level change*: Theories in this area explain the importance of
  full community participation, community capacity building, community
  development and community empowerment. In this model these
  approaches are understood as community organization strategies in
  which there is an agenda for change.
♦ *Environmental level change*: External sources of community change may be
  understood in terms of national norms (e.g., secular trends), economic
  theories and social movements. Such changes may include the effects of
  government policy and laws.

The depiction of the whole model shows how each level from the external
environment, down through community groups and partnerships to organizations and social networks, impacts on changes in individual behaviours
(with interactions at each level). Thompson and Kinne use the example of
an antismoking intervention (COMMIT) to illustrate how social movements, changing norms and government policy on smoking impacted on
and encouraged community involvement through community organizations, commercial organizations, health systems and social networks. These
changes influence the formation of action groups (such as DARE, Wellness
Groups, schools) to directly influence individuals' attitudes and hence their
behaviour.

Several other integrated models of health determining conditions in general, rather than behaviour in particular, have been developed. For example,
the model first proposed by Dahlgren and Whitehead (1991) as an approach
to inequalities in health has been extremely influential in public health
discourse. In this model, individual characteristics such as age, gender and
heredity are understood to be nested within successive layers of influence
on health: lifestyle, social and community factors, and living and working
conditions. These are overarched by general socioeconomic, cultural and
environmental effects. A version of this sort of model, incorporating social
theory to explain some relationships within the model, has been developed

by Labonte and colleagues (2002) to inform the population health research work of a multidisciplinary unit. This model (see Figure 6.1) includes the understanding that the ecosystem and the health of the planet is of overarching importance to health. The graphic version of the model has also been drawn to emphasis that each level is understood, not only as a separate layer of influence on health, but also as affecting every other layer or band. Such models have been influential and helpful in guiding public health research, strategies, and policy making over the last two decades.

Multilevel programmes

Social ecological models suggest the importance of multilevel interventions, that is, interventions that are working at several levels of the ecological system at the same time. One of the important effects of shifts towards ecological models has been the development of large scale intervention 'programmes' designed to influence change at the interpersonal, organizational, community and policy levels. Stokols (1992) emphasized that the social-ecological perspective demands multilevel interventions that combine complementary behavioural and environmental changes. For example, behaviour modification programmes for smoking cessation (such as 'quitting programmes' or media advertising) may be more effective if they coincide with no smoking policies in workplaces and laws that prohibit

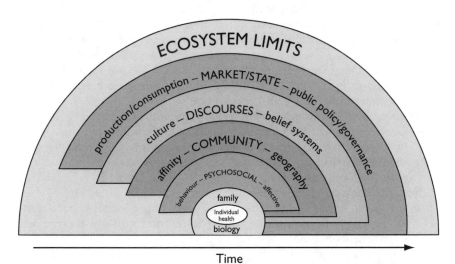

Figure 6.1 Saskatchewan Population Health and Evaluation Research Unit (SPHERU) conceptual model of health determining conditions

Source: From Labonte et al., 2002; reproduced with the permission of the Minister of Public Works and Government Services Canada, 2008.

smoking in public places. It is also important that influential levels of the social environment (e.g., workplace managers, politicians, media promoters, movie stars) are reinforcing the same message and not contradicting each other. Merzel and D'Affliti (2003) describe how community-based prevention programmes should be integrated and comprehensive (rather than limited to one setting such as medical care) and systematically involve community leaders, social networks, mass communication campaigns and direct education of the general population. 'Community-based programs use multiple interventions, targeting change among individuals, groups, and organizations, and they often incorporate strategies to create policy and environmental changes' (p. 558).

In regard to exercise, Sallis et al. (2006) have made a very strong call for the implementation of multilevel interventions based on ecological models using multidisciplinary teams. They propose a complex but practical model (focused on the physical environment) in which the person is the centre of surrounding levels of influence including their perceived environment, the active living domain (behaviour), the settings for behaviour and the policy environment. The level of the active living domain is at the heart of their proposed agenda which focuses on changes in active recreation, active transport, occupational activities and household activities. To implement these changes, their model suggests the need to target individuals, social environments, physical environments and public policy.

Merzel and D'Affliti (2003) have reviewed many examples of multilevel programmes in the US that address a range of issues. Two examples from their overview of such interventions are noted here to indicate the sort of activities that are typically included in such large scale programmes:

1 The Pawtucket Heart Health Program.
   ♦ *Individual level*: Adult education programmes; self-help materials; screening; counselling; and referral events.
   ♦ *Group level*: Lay volunteers to deliver group interventions.
   ♦ *Community level*: Restaurant menu labelling; supermarket shelf labelling; food providers and workplace cafeterias offering heart friendly menus; installation of exercise facilities; community-wide contests; mass media advertising.
2 Fighting Back (substance abuse programme).
   ♦ *Individual level*: Youth self-esteem programmes; after-school programmes; youth mentoring; youth job referral; drop-out preventions; treatment services.
   ♦ *Group level*: Parenting classes; workplace programmes; training of health professionals.
   ♦ *Community level*: Community organizing; community policing; neighbourhood drug clean-ups; increasing alcohol tax; banning Sunday liquor sales; limiting youth access to alcohol.

As you may imagine, it is very easy to suggest multilevel interventions in theory, and much more expensive and more difficult to implement them in practice. Several authors have begun to grapple with these issues. Chappell et al. (2005) suggest that many health promotion programmes remain level specific and are still largely focused on change at the individual level, owing to the difficulties of implementing multilevel health promotion. They suggested new strategies for ensuring a multilevel focus, including using multiple methods for community assessment and assessing project activities according to the levels at which change is required. They describe how these strategies were used in implementing a neighbourhood health development programme to prevent type 2 diabetes. Using a social-ecological model, the programme developers were committed to change at multiple levels. In their example, the strategies were successfully used to move from micro to the inclusion of more macro municipal policy levels of action. Maclean et al. (2007) have reported on the practical difficulties of managing a complex multidisciplinary intervention that was designed to promote tobacco free living among young adults aged 18 to 25 years. They describe several challenges (as well as successes) and suggest the need for increased understandings of how adding levels of intervention and including a wide range of team members overloads collaborative systems.

Issues in using social ecological models

The social ecological models are based in a positivist epistemology with the associated values of objectivity, value neutrality and control. Programmes that draw upon social-ecological models remain focused on changing individual behaviours while taking into account the important influence of the environment. The issues of behavioural risks focus the attention of programme designers so that, although systems theories include conceptions of the environmental levels as interdependent with reciprocal influences, in health promotion practice such models tend to remain focused on individual behaviour change as the outcome. The language of these programmes suggest that rational choice is still seen as the basis of health behaviour, but the physical and social environment are constraints on the correct choices. The environment is thus seen largely as a constraint or influence on individually based action or health outcomes whose aims have been predetermined.

There are some problems inherent in the use of such models. Although increasing numbers of public health researchers endorse a comprehensive approach and many practitioners base their work on a social ecological model there are no clear explanations of how the different levels of actions connect with each other and include health. The integrated models available are not well suited for use of systems theories to explain the linkages, and much work still tends to focus on separate levels of action (even if they are in operation together). For example, there has been a great deal of success in using multilevel approaches to reducing cigarette smoking and it has been well recognized that environmental influences have had a lot to do with the changes in smoking behaviour over the last 50 years. However, the models developed in antitobacco use campaigns have not transferred successfully to application in diet and exercise interventions. There is a need for better understanding of how the social environment actually functions. McLeroy et al. (2003) have joined the many recent calls to develop better theories of community change that take into account the organizational, community, environmental and policy level relationships and feed-back loops of a social ecology.

Cornish (2004) also noted that there are few models that can be used to link individual health with community contexts. She has made an important move with a pragmatist approach to conceptualize health related behaviour. Beginning with Bronfenbrenner's ecological model, she includes dialogical theorizing to explain the concept of 'mediating moments'. In Cornish's examples, the condom use of sex workers in a Calcutta red light district is examined in particular moments in which the social-environmental factors become salient and concrete. Thus, there are particular moments when social factors, such as time pressure, fear of losing earnings, unity, poverty, male demands and exploitation of women, materially affect the women's opportunities to use condoms.

Social determinants of health

Some models for health promotion have drawn on more highly developed theories of the social determinants of health. Many of these approaches have developed along with the concern to understand inequalities in health. Accordingly these models draw on theories that explain health related behaviour as constructed by social, cultural, economic and political conditions, and health differentials as the result of social inequalities and injustice. The use of these approaches is part of a shift away from problem-based theories of health behaviour to conceptions of socially based health promotion and a concern with the development of resilience rather than illness prevention. These theories have been used in the development of participatory models of community development that include the importance of concepts such as empowerment, capacity building and partnerships.

Participation

Participatory approaches to community health promotion include understandings of the importance of participation by members of any community in any activities related to their well being. 'Participation' is an everyday word which has had a particular meaning in community development contexts for some time. Heller et al. (1984) defined citizen participation as '. . . a process in which individuals take part in decision making in the institutions, programs, and environments that affect them' (p. 339). According to these authors, advocates argue that citizen participation gives individuals a sense of control (important in itself to health) and enables people's needs and values to be taken into account.

Community-based participatory approaches to intervention include social and cultural understandings of community and are based on principles of collaboration. Hence, 'participation' by community members in programmes and services to enhance their health is an appealing concept. The notion of participation in health promotion is supported by the World Health Organization, and statements such as: 'engaging local communities to participate in identifying their own health priorities spurs the development of innovatory culturally acceptable solutions with locally available resources' (Paul, 2004) are encouragingly positive. According to Dinham (2005), 'local participation is regarded as axiomatic' in community development approaches, both as a necessary condition for change, and in terms of the values of empowerment and partnership (p. 3). There is a wealth of information available regarding participatory approaches. For example, an excellent website with many links to such resources, including different languages, is at: http://depts.washington.edu/ccph/commbas.html For another model of participation with a participatory research and empowerment focus you may be more interested in the Participatory Action Research models covered in Chapter 5. Here, I will focus on some of the important concepts that are, as suggested by Dinham, part of the participatory approach: empowerment, capacity building and partnerships.

Empowerment

The concept of empowerment has long been an important aim of those working toward community participation in many settings. Alexis de Tocqueville argued in 1830 that citizens were being isolated by the growth of cities and the scope of societies, and that they could overcome the resulting sense of powerlessness only through active involvement in common concerns (Heller et al., 1984). Participation in community activities is still seen as a way for people to gain some control of their environment and their health. Laverack (2007) focuses his model of participatory health promotion practice on this concept of empowerment ('building empowered communities' is the subtitle of his book). Participation is of no benefit to community members unless it includes control and power over the activities and outcomes. Laverack describes community empowerment as involving a struggle to gain power from others, and '. . . a process by which communities gain more control over the decisions and resources that influence their lives, including the determinants of health' (p. 29). Laverack's model of community-based interaction is a ladder on the lowest rungs of which are aspects of participation leading towards the highest rungs of empowerment.

In this model, the outcomes of empowered social and political action are understood as the determinants of health. Much empowerment intervention work has been focused on socially excluded populations such as minority ethnicities, women, youth and the poor. Interventions aimed at empowering women, youth and chronic disease sufferers have shown improvements in many aspects of well being (Wallerstein, 2006).

Gaining power involves a struggle with those who hold power and if we do not include understandings of dominant norms and social practices that reproduce power relations, then the very discourse and practices of 'empowerment' may be damaging. Petersen and Lupton (1996) use post-structuralist theory to critique the 'new public health' in terms of power relations. They have shown how 'participation' and 'empowerment' is part of a 'duties discourse' which uses the appealing language of new social movements to transform people's awareness so they become more self-regulating, while serving the goals of the State and other agencies. Ramella and De la Cruz (2000) include this critique in their understanding of participation, but they also note that this theoretical approach only allows for a discourse of resistance; it does not help us to understand how to move towards empowered social and political action. To move beyond the post-structuralist account of power relations (which is revealing but not a model for practice), and to include the possibility for critical social action they draw on Habermas and the critical theory of Freire to conceptualize participation as communication and intersubjective action (as opposed to the behaviour of an individual rational subject) that is oriented towards mutual understanding. In practice this means that everyday life is discussed, problems and power relations (which may have been taken for granted) are highlighted, and plans for addressing problems are developed in participatory dialogue between teachers and students, or health professionals and community members. Ramella and De la Cruz describe the application of this approach to adolescent sexual health promotion in Peru through social clubs organized by and for young people. Guareschi and Jovchelovitch (2004) similarly draw on the Freirian concepts of dialogue and conscientization to highlight the social psychological dimensions of participation and its role in health promotion. Their intervention in Brazil is described in more detail in Chapter 7. The use of critical theory highlights the political and ideological basis of empowerment and participatory approaches which are often unacknowledged.

Capacity building and resilience

Laverack's (2007) ladder of community-based interaction begins with community readiness and culminates in community empowerment. In this model, communities participate and develop community capacity along the road to taking action. In other words, communities must develop the skills, organizing abilities and resources that will enable them to act. Labonte and Laverack (2001) describe several different uses of the term 'capacity building' in the literature. They also suggest that the terms 'community development', 'empowerment', 'social capital' and 'social cohesion' have been used for similar things. All this is very confusing and points to the lack of good theory in these areas of health promotion. However, for practical uses they suggest several domains of community capacity which are important for health promotion programmes. The areas are: participation, leadership, organizational structures, problem assessment, 'asking why' (critical assessment of problems), resource mobilization, links with others, roles of outside agents and programme management. These authors also suggest that only particular domains fit particular situations and the assessment of capacity is a very practical issue. Many practitioners assess the capacities to be developed (e.g., research skills, leadership skills, funding application skills) according to the needs of the programme (which suggests a need for ongoing and rigorous reflexivity on the part of programme coordinators).

Raeburn et al. (2006) have provided five case studies of successful capacity building projects for health promotion from different parts of the world, including:

♦ Community directed treatment and monitoring of river blindness in 19 countries in Africa.
♦ The participatory budget process in Peru which allows citizens to debate and set municipal investment priorities.
♦ Poor rural communities in Honduras initiated the task of establishing and running their own health clinic, supported by the Ministry of Health.
♦ A low income suburban community and a university in New Zealand collaborated to develop a community house to enhance community well being. This project survives 30 years later and meets many community needs.
♦ Farmers in a poverty stricken rural community in Thailand reassessed the concept of farming for money and now pursue physical and mental health. They have rebuilt their way of life and with an NGO have developed a network to share their community development skills.

The concept of capacity building does accord with the shift to notions of resilience. Raeburn et al. (2006) suggest that as a part of a tradition of community action in health promotion, capacity building models reflect the shift to notions of assets and strengths as opposed to pathology and deficiency models. Antonovsky (1996) proposed what has become a very influential model of salutogenesis to guide these aspects of health promotion. McCreanor and Watson (2004) have used this theory as a basis to suggest that social connection is a critical resilience capacity for health. They conceptualize connection as the links with others and suggest that this social feature of the environment has already been shown in the literature to be an important health protective factor. These authors were considering the mental health of young people, but the resilience capacity of social connections is one of the most well known contributors to the well being of individuals (when conceptualized as social support and social networks) or of communities (as social capital).

One area in which these concepts have been applied is the development of community arts projects. The salutogenic effects, on individual and community health, of participation in the arts are increasingly recognized. Health promotion practitioners are recognizing the capacity building power of community arts programmes as ways '. . . to celebrate community strengths, assets, and connections' (Carson et al., 2006). This resilience-based approach draws upon the existing talents of community members, and develops opportunities for social connections, expression and sharing of ideas and opportunities for creative dialogue. In Canada, a community arts-based programme was initiated to use local strengths to develop a safety culture (Murray and Tilley, 2006; see Chapter 7). In the UK, an arts centre was developed as a community-based initiative within a broader health promotion project (Carson et al., 2006). In addition to providing health promoting activities and the development of social support, the arts centre was seen to build community strength as an end in itself by developing the community's own strengths and assets. In the US, Stephenson (2007) describes the use of a social network model to underpin the development of a community arts programme in a threatened and disintegrating community. The aims of the programme were to build social capital and provide opportunities for an arts-based civic dialogue, stimulate community conversation, reflection and change by using the existing energy and motivation of local arts organizations and leadership. These same ideas have been applied to developments of the physical environment. Semenza and Krishnasamy (2007) describe a health promoting neighbourhood intervention in which residents of urban communities were involved in planning, designing and developing aesthetic improvements to their streets and malls. These included street murals, gardens, fountains and benches. The project was intended to strengthen social networks and social capital by involving the citizens and providing places in their neighbourhoods that would meet their own needs.

Partnerships

Capacity has been identified as emerging in four areas of community coalitions: within members, relationships, organizations and within programmes (Wells et al., 2007). Each of these areas is an important aspect of the partnerships that are formed to develop community based programmes. The partnerships that are formed between local citizens, scientists, health practitioners, local and government bodies, and organizations such as universities and health funders are critical to the success of health promotion activities and the source of shared capacity. Laverack (2007) notes the importance for example, of the different sorts of experience and skills (e.g., research skills from the university; medical knowledge from health practitioners; and local cultural and practical knowledge from community members) that different partners bring to any programme.

Partnerships are also increasingly recognized as a source of problematic relationships and unequal power sharing. For example, it has proved difficult for some health professionals to give up their status as experts in community settings (see Guareschi and Jovchelovitch, 2004; Wallerstein, 2006; Campbell et al., 2007). Thus, such partnerships have become an object of study and critique themselves. Matheson et al. (2005) reviewed this literature and suggested that to address complex social problems, such as reducing health inequalities, the theory and practice of partnership approaches must be addressed much more carefully. In an example of the sort of findings of such study, Campbell et al. (2004) used social theory to show how 'partnerships' between members of different social groups (in their example African-Caribbean community members, voluntary group members and local councils in the UK) can be counter-productive. They suggest that deprived minority groups lack the bonding and bridging social capital to participate effectively in such partnerships, which are in danger of simply reproducing pre-existing power relations and social inequalities.

Issues in participatory approaches

The values behind most participatory models include collaboration, empowerment and political equality. As appealing as they sound, partnerships between community residents and service providers have not been easy to achieve, and there have been many problems with the implementation of what has turned out to be another of those attractive and popular, yet broad and undertheorized, concepts. There is already an extensive literature exploring the problems and obstacles in participatory approaches. Here, I note two broad approaches that have been used recently to address problems.

The first broad approach has been to describe the very practical problems, along with the achievements, associated with encouraging participation in health promotion programmes. The response to this way of understanding the issues is to describe the barriers as experienced and to provide suggestions for overcoming them. For example, Nelson et al. (2004) describe the successes and difficulties of involving the residents of a Canadian community in a health promotion programme for families. They note the barriers to participation in their programme, which included language and cultural barriers, financial barriers, work overload and people's resistance to the involvement of professionals or schools and to engaging in formal meetings. Similarly, Whitehead et al. (2005) have described the barriers to involving youth in South Africa. These sorts of approaches generally accept the notion of participation as beneficial. However, as noted by Mukherjea (2006) the ostensibly democratic approach to community empowerment ignores detrimental power imbalances. The external organizers themselves have greater privilege and attach more status to their knowledge, which affect their roles in the community and make it difficult for community members to question them. In general, participatory interventions have been subjected to considerable critique regarding the non-representativeness of participants and exclusion of many community members (e.g., Robertson and Minkler, 1994), the dangers of non-reflexive practice in which dominant norms of participation that advantage powerful groups go unchallenged (e.g., Petersen and Lupton, 1996; Wakefield and Poland, 2005), and the potential for participation to relieve the state of responsibility, and for community members to be blamed for their failure to participate (e.g., Dinham, 2005). In the early 1990s commentators were noting that empowerment had become a 'buzzword' appropriated for strategic use by the powerful (Guttman, 2000).

A second approach, often in the light of these critiques, is to discuss the problems and complexities of participation in health promotion and community development in principle. Hence, various approaches to the nature and meaning of participation have been described, and several typologies developed in attempts to explore and define the different practices, aims, and ideologies behind community development activities. For example, Arnstein (1971) classically described 'eight rungs' on a ladder of community participation ranging from token consultation by outsiders, to complete citizen control of a programme of change. Popple (1995) contributed a typology which identifies a spectrum of participatory intervention ranging from consensus to radicalism. Morgan (2001) contrasted two different perspectives: the utilitarian (aiming for success by utilizing local resources) and empowerment approaches (aiming to change power structures and allow for participation of excluded communities). Such definitions have been useful as the basis for critical reflection on the aims and practices of community development workers, but as explanations of the nature of participation as a social practice, they fall short. As Guareschi and Jovchelovitch (2004) say: 'In real settings participation is messy, takes time, and escapes neat definitions' (p. 313). This suggests that we need broader theorizing that can account for the issues, whatever the approach taken in the field, and help us to understand what it means to participate; why people would participate in any particular activity; and in whose interests they participate. Thus, a third approach is to develop broader social psychological conceptualizations of participation which are located in the practicalities, purposes and power relations of social life.

A social psychological model of participation

Campbell and Jovchelovitch (2000) proposed a model toward a social psychology of participation to guide practice in reducing health inequalities. They argued that the key constituents of community are only enacted in participation. Furthermore, the formation, enactment and transformation of community in participatory activities is based on three key concepts:

♦ *Identity*. Social identity plays a key role in understanding the formation of any community. The key component of any community is a shared identity. Freire's notion of conscientization explains how at particular moments members of socially excluded groupings may challenge their marginalized identity and construct new identities (thus 'prostitutes' become 'sex workers').

♦ *Social representations*. Social representations theory has provided a way of understanding local knowledge. Practical and symbolic resources of particular social groups must be recognized but not necessarily idealized (thus representations of masculinity and men as risk takers are counterproductive in HIV/AIDS prevention work).

♦ *Power*. An understanding of power relations is essential to understanding the conditions under which participation is enacted. Bourdieu's theory of practice provides a useful way of understanding the struggles for power between groups and the access to use of economic, social and symbolic resources (capitals) that are enacted even within health promotion projects.

Campbell (2003) has developed this framework and particularly the use of Bourdieu's critical conceptualization of social capital. She has used this social psychological model to inform our understandings of what empowerment and participation mean for disadvantaged groups (in her examples, poor mine workers, sex workers and youth at risk for HIV/AIDS in South Africa). In unequal societies, social capital may be used by advantaged groups to further exclude those with low social status. Campbell also discusses how partnerships are difficult to foster when 'communities may often be strongly divided by power differentials, radically different world views and high levels of mistrust' (p. 166). This conceptualization has been used to explain why many participatory community projects do not achieve their aims, despite the best intentions of the organizers and partners in such projects. Campbell's framework also provides a model for considering community participation which provides possibilities for deprived people to gain more control over their lives and health, while taking account of the importance of the broader structural and political forces which shape people's lives.

Cultural and local models of health

If people in a community are working from different cultural models of health and social life than those of the health practitioners who are interested in partnership, then there is an extra layer of negotiation to include in developing a model for any intervention. There is a great deal of anthropological and sociological work for health practitioners to draw upon as a start to understanding the differences in priorities and expectations that must arise in these situations. Labonte et al. (2005) described some of these difficulties for the members of research teams comprising Western and First Nations people in Canada, and the notion of an 'ethical space' in which different world views may be exchanged and interpretations negotiated.

Whare Tapa Wha

In New Zealand both Māori and European practitioners may draw on the models developed by Māori researchers. The most well known of these has been provided by Professor Mason Durie (a Māori academic and author) who has drawn upon Māori culture and his professional knowledge of public health issues to develop two models for health and health promotion. *Whare Tapa Wha* (described in Chapter 4) makes instant sense to New Zealand health practitioners and is widely used in practice in areas of health promotion such as chronic disease care, drug and alcohol use, and smoking programmes with Māori. Glover (2005) describes the detailed application of this model to Māori experiences of smoking, and its use as the basis of a holistic intervention programme for Māori. In general, the principles of *Whare Tapa Wha* mean that the wider aspects of community life are included in interventions so that family (*whanau*) is understood as an important aspect of any treatment or intervention, clinics and smoke free programmes are located in more culturally relevant places such as on local *marae*, and broader activities such as the development of sports teams and events are included in programmes to develop health.

Te Pae Mahutonga

Durie (1999) has developed a model specifically to guide health promotion practice. Like *Whare Tapa Wha*, this model is based on a powerful metaphor that includes important symbols of identity. This is *Te Pae Mahutonga* (the Southern Cross constellation) which has been used as a navigational aid and is closely associated with the discovery of Aotearoa by Polynesian navigators and later by Europeans. The model includes six key aspects. First the four stars of *Te Pae Mahutonga* represent:

♦ *Mauriora*: Inner strength, vitality which depend on secure cultural identity and access to the Māori world. A goal of health promotion then is to promote the security of this identity.
♦ *Waiora*: The connection of human wellness with the cosmic, terrestrial and water environments. Good health depends on access to a healthy and unpolluted environment.
♦ *Toiora*: Healthy lifestyles and personal behaviours, which include good

nutrition, and avoiding alcohol and drugs, tobacco use and unsafe driving practices.

♦ *Te Oranga*: Participation in society. This means full and equal opportunity for participation including access to employment, goods and services, schools, health services, and sport and recreation activities of choice.

The fifth and sixth elements are represented by the two 'pointers' that are a part of this constellation:

♦ *Nga Manukura*: Leadership from within the Māori community and development of a skilled health promotion work force.
♦ *Te Mana Whakahaere*: Autonomy, ownership and control by communities that must be provided by the appropriate legislative and policy environment.

Durie has developed this model (and work based on it) from the original understandings of Sir Maui Pomare, a prominent Māori public health practitioner and influential minister of health throughout the last century. Durie's development of Pomare's recognition of key aspects has also been influenced by the Ottawa charter. In many ways the vision of these leaders, who have been working closely with the health issues for Māori, may be seen as paralleled by recent developments in health promotion practice internationally. The growing understandings of the importance of the whole environment, the recognition of the impact of social disparities and exclusion, and the importance for health of participation, control and capacity are reflected in these culturally specific models.

Health promotion messages and the media

Public health messages disseminated through the media are often just one aspect of broader multilevel programmes. However, these messages are a commonly used method for persuading people to change their health related behaviour in some way, and are often taken for granted as a medium for educating populations about certain issues. Attempts to change the social environment are often conducted through or with the assistance of media campaigns and health communication campaigns are increasingly recognized as social actions in their own right (Cho and Salmon, 2007). Thus, there is a great deal of theorizing available to assist health promoters to understand the potential impact of their messages (for good or for harm) and such messages are so ubiquitous that they deserve a section to themselves in this chapter.

Social marketing

One popular model for health communications is social marketing (Hastings and McDermott, 2006). Many countries, including Australia, New Zealand, Canada and the US have social marketing facilities as part of their health services. Members of the public in these and many other countries are familiar with the sorts of media health campaigns that result from this interest. Social marketing has been developed using the tools of persuasion that have been developed by commercial advertisers. It is now understood that the wider environment including health care infrastructure, the physical environment, and social policy changes must support these campaigns if they are to have the desired impact. Nevertheless, although the approach is called 'social', it is theoretically aimed at the individual and the stated aims are to change people's (albeit in large numbers) attitudes, intentions and behaviours (and perhaps lead them to persuade others, see Hastings and McDermott, 2006).

Community radio

In line with the principles of participation, community radio is emerging as a medium that may be used to promote health while shifting power and capacity back to the community. There are now numerous examples of how community radio stations have been used to contribute to the health and social development of communities (Pepall et al., 2007). Radio is the chosen medium because it is affordable for low income groups; relevant for people who have low literacy; and accessible by community members who may produce and broadcast culturally relevant information. However, such efforts are always in danger, as in other participatory approaches, of being hijacked by more powerful or articulate groups, or of doing unanticipated and unintentional harm without good theory to guide reflexive practice.

A model of the effects of communication

Cho and Salmon (2007) conceptualize media campaigns as social actions in which different values and interests of those with different levels of power compete for influence. They systematically describe the conceptual dimensions and types of unintended effects of such campaigns in a framework intended to contribute to the development of theory and practice of health communication campaigns. The intended and unintended effects of media messages have long been considered in communication theories, ranging from 'noise' in mathematical models to recognition of the 'boomerang' effects of fear appeals and the notion of psychological reactance. Such theorizing operates at the individual level effects of specific content, while Cho and Salmon wish to include understandings of the broader social effects of messages: campaigns aimed at changes in individuals may modify the systems, values and cultures of a community, and these are beyond the traditional bounds of enquiry. Their detailed typology of 11 dimensions of unintended effects accounts for: individual and social effects, short- and long-term effects, intended and unintended audiences, specific and diffusive content, and desirable or undesirable effects. (Of course, the latter in particular will also depend upon the values of the message proponents, see Guttman, 2000). Cho and Salmon (2007) hope that their typology will lead to investigation and refinement of the theoretical framework. One area of theorizing that already takes into account the very social nature of communications is media studies.

Media theories

Recent media theorizing provides some useful ways to understand the effect of media health messages. The first important point to be made is that today most of the world's citizens live in 'mediated' societies in which the press, television, radio and the Internet are involved in the general circulation of ideas in social life. The myths, vocabularies and social representations with which we construct our world and practice are no longer those of small communities. Rather, they are mediated interactions with characters in popular culture with whom we share the symbolic resources of social construction along with our friends and families (Hodgetts et al., 2005). Late modern societies are saturated with media messages (Silverstone, 1999) which include frameworks for understanding health issues. People do not need to actually hear specific media messages for them to enter their lives. Once entered into social dialogue, media representations take on a life of their own: they are appropriated and recirculated. Thus, the conceptualization of health messages as discrete fragments that are taken up by individuals and acted upon within a limited time frame does not represent what actually occurs. There are two main threads of media theory that can help us to examine the life of media messages.

First, theories that explain mediation as an ongoing and interactive aspect of social life. It is not a linear process through which media messages and values are simply imposed on the public. Gerbner's cultivation theory (see Gerbner et al., 1994) proposes that the influence of the media is derived from a total pattern of coverage of certain norms and values. It describes the ways in which people from particular social milieu are more or less likely to be drawn toward the norms and values included in particular messages. The development of these norms and values occurs across time through a dialogical process in which public opinion is both drawn upon and shaped.

Second, to explain the active role of the audiences in this process, Couldry (2003) proposes that we pay attention to the ritual dimensions of media communication. These rituals include practices such as discussing health information from a website or magazine, or banning smoking in the home. Such approaches describe the development of shared norms and values through the media's roles in providing shared spaces and routine practices that foster a sense of belonging and participation. The media allows us to share ideas and concerns beyond our everyday practices. Thus, the media cultivate a sense of shared space and vocabulary for understanding health and participating in social life (Hodgetts et al., 2005). This appropriation also includes resistance and reshaping as illustrated by Crossley's (2004) example of gay men who deliberately participate in sexual practices that have been deemed 'unsafe' through media messages.

Such complex theories of mediated social life support suggestions, such as those of Wallack (2003), for more socially oriented approaches to uses of media to support social justice and the development of social capital. Wallack describes the potential of approaches such as civic journalism, media advocacy and photovoice. The goal of these approaches, like community radio mentioned above, is to engage people in deliberation of problems, discussions of solutions and participation in the processes of social and political change. These are media for giving a voice rather than leaving a message (p. 616) and such approaches are based on the understanding that community life is mediated and shared.

Addressing structural and political issues

The models reviewed above reflect some serious shifts toward ecological and participatory models for health promotion. These models include considerations of the person's physical and social environment (albeit in different ways), and levels of power including personal, community, institutional and State power to shape people's lives and health. Some approaches are based on addressing the broader causes of health inequalities at the level of influencing social policy and the structure of society that is understood as perpetuating and worsening those inequalities. Within these broad aims some approaches to guide practical intervention that will change inequalities in health have arisen. Lifecourse, physical environment, social policy and social justice approaches may all be seen as contributing to a concern to specifically address health inequalities.

Lifecourse approach

To address inequalities directly, many authors suggest a broad front for action (driven by social policy), which includes improved living and working conditions across the lifecourse to include early child development, education and support for older individuals. The 'lifecourse approach' is a framework for conceptualizing the complexity of factors that influence health inequalities. As such, it acknowledges the influence of socioeconomic structure (labour market, welfare policies), material factors (housing, living standards, environmental hazards), social networks and relationships (family functioning, peer support) behavioural influences (smoking, nutrition), and psychosocial factors (parental divorce, transition) (Earl and National Health Committee, 2002). It values changing unequal conditions and supporting those affected by inequalities at particularly vulnerable times of life. Epidemiological evidence is used to support the life stage approach. For example, Davey Smith et al. (2001) reported on a longitudinal study of university graduates which shows that, among a group of men who were in similarly advantaged social circumstances in their adult life, those who came from more disadvantaged childhood backgrounds were more likely to die of CHD earlier.

This evidence may be interpreted in a number of ways and within a life stage approach there are several different models which specify points for health promotion intervention (Earl and National Health Committee, 2002):

♦ Pathway models suggest that circumstances in early life influence the pathway to adult health. Thus poor childhood conditions influence trajectories into and through adulthood.
♦ Critical periods models identify sensitive periods of development. The evidence for these models tends to focus on childhood and suggests exposure to deprivation in early life has long-term health effects. This model highlights the importance of parental influences, particularly maternal (including prenatal) influences.
♦ Accumulation models hypothesize that exposure to disadvantage at different life stages has a chronic and cumulative effect on health. They draw on evidence to suggest that poor circumstances throughout life confer the greatest risk of poor health. There is also an understanding that poor circumstances at one life stage can be mitigated by better circumstances at another which supports the usefulness of intervention at several stages across the lifecourse.

In general, a life stage approach is based on the understanding that interventions have cohort, age and time effects, and that there are critical phases or transitions in the lifecourse when the impact will be particularly far reaching (Whitehead, 2007). The different models suggest particularly sensitive times for intervention. For example, there are several early childhood programmes aimed at providing social support for parents and early educational advantages for children.

Environment

Housing is an example of an area in which evidence is being gathered specifically with the aim of influencing government policy in areas that contribute to unequal material conditions and unequal health outcomes. An overview of urban planning policy in the US (Mueller and Tighe, 2007) shows that in the past there were understandings that poor housing conditions are detrimental to the whole community; at one time connections were clearly seen between housing, health and social well being. More recently, these connections have become less apparent and there are tensions for urban planners based on conflicts between the needs of low income families to live in affordable housing, and the needs of the middle class to retain property values as housing has become an important and increasingly expensive commodity. These tensions which are evident in many parts of the world today, place the issue of housing at the heart of the social causes of inequalities in health. There is evidence that quality of housing is related directly to health, but this evidence must be re-established to persuade policy analysts that good housing is an issue for health. The UK government's Wanless report of 2004 examined the cost effectiveness of taking action to improve the health of the whole population and to reduce health inequalities. This report highlighted lack of evidence for the cost effectiveness of public health and social interventions, and identified the need to collect better evidence of the effects of interventions in the housing sector (Thomson and Petticrew, 2007).

One study seen as contributing to this sort of evidence is a longitudinal intervention conducted in New Zealand. Howden–Chapman et al. (2007) showed that across seven low income communities improvements in insulation led to warmer houses and improved respiratory health. Their conclusions are that 'fitting insulation is a cost effective intervention for improving health and wellbeing. It has a high degree of acceptance by the community, policy makers, and politicians' (p. 463). Thus, there is a growing acceptance by governments (Sweden and the Netherlands apparently leading the way in this approach to policy) that other traditional areas of state policy such as housing, environment, transport and education are directly related to health, and there is a growing role for health promoters at this policy level.

Social policy action

Based on the growing weight of epidemiological evidence for a gradient in health, Marmot (1999) suggested a focus on building equality in the degree of autonomy and participation for all members of society. Marmot (2004) further suggested that these changes to the social environment across a broad front require the attention of policymakers and lobbying by health professionals. Raphael (2000), on considering the evidence for the growing social causes of health inequalities suggested some specific courses of action for public health workers in Canada including: developing communication between various sectors concerned with economic inequality; using the media to educate the public about the consequences of increasing economic inequality and poverty for health; lobbying local health departments; and lobbying governments to maintain the community and service structures that help to maintain health and well being. Exactly these kinds of actions have been practised in Europe since the 1990s. Countries such as the Netherlands, Sweden and Spain were the first to put health inequalities on health policy agendas, and Moss (2003) describes how public action in the European Union has identified inequalities as a priority area. Much of this has been due to media attention and public awareness of the issues, and a steady stream of reports and prestigious scientific publications (such as the work of Wilkinson and Marmot and colleagues), and networking across sectors as suggested by Raphael (2000). Thus, a growing number of countries are now devising policies and interventions to address inequalities (although there remains a paucity of theory and models of causation on which to base policies and interventions, see Exworthy et al., 2006; Whitehead, 2007).

Marmot, Raphael and Moss were calling health promotion attention to the understanding that research findings do not automatically lead to changes in policy or practice. There is strong awareness of the need for concerted and systematic approaches to policy advocacy in public health circles. Brownson et al. (2006) note that 'practitioners working in government agencies have to learn how to influence policy development without direct lobbying. This often involves working in coalitions that can mobilize support and advocate for specific issues' (p. 361). Felix (2007) describes a policy streams model to explain how issues may influence policy. In this model, changes in a problem stream (evidence and awareness), policy stream (possible solutions), and political stream (public and politician's mood and attitudes) come together at a point called the 'policy window' (the opportunity for policy adoption), with the aid of a policy entrepreneur who is the advocate.

In regard to the problem and policy streams, Brownson et al. (2006), reviewed environmental and policy approaches to the prevention of chronic disease. They provide a conceptual framework for understanding the effects of these approaches which include successful policy interventions to alter the physical, economic and communication environment. These domains are applicable to many public health issues, but the authors also note that, although such interventions have the potential to equalize the environment, the evidence to date does not apply to populations with large health inequalities. Flisher et al. (2007) describe a new project to study mental health policy development in four African countries (Ghana, South Africa, Uganda and Zambia) which does have a focus on inequity. The purpose of the project is to provide new knowledge regarding comprehensive and inclusive multisectoral approaches to changing the negative relationship between poverty, exclusion and mental health. These authors begin with a complex conceptual framework for the development of policy and assessment of its effectiveness on this basis.

Social justice

Having inequalities on the public health policy agenda is only the first step in addressing the issues. There is much work to be done by health promoters in developing models for intervention in this recently highlighted area of concern. Whitehead (2007) has overviewed actions taken to tackle social inequalities in health that are supported by government policies and these range from the approaches at the individual, through community, environmental, to macro political changes.

Proponents of social justice claim that it is at this latter level of macro political change that health promotion efforts will be most fruitful. We need clear understandings of the mundane political conflicts and the struggles of everyday life between different groups to explain why some groups are healthier than others (Hofrichter, 2003). Beauchamp (2003) states that 'public health should be a way of doing justice . . .' (p. 276). By this he means that health must be seen as the responsibility of the whole society, and public health ethical activity must necessarily challenge the norms of 'market-justice'. In challenging the effects of the ethics of capitalism on public health, Levins (2003) further suggests that health must be seen as a class struggle. Unless the underlying power issues are challenged, the policies developed by government institutions often reflect the interests of the powerful whose focus is on profit. Those policies, ostensibly aimed at improving people's lives, are often 'hobbled' by systematic restraints and hidden barriers that serve these powerful interests.

Lynch et al. (2000) have similarly argued that income or status inequalities are a reflection of structural issues in society that are affecting population health through a complex matrix of resulting material conditions. These conditions are seen as:

> . . . a combination of negative exposures and lack of resources held by individuals, along with systematic underinvestment across a wide range of human, physical, health, and social infrastructure. An unequal income distribution is one result of historical, cultural, and political-economic processes. These processes influence the private resources available to individuals and shape the nature of public infrastructure – education, health services, transportation, environmental controls, availability of food, quality of housing, occupational health regulations – that form the 'neo-material' matrix of contemporary life.
>
> (p. 320)

Social justice approaches suggest that health promoters must go beyond ameliorative public health measures to those that focus on the causes of economic and social inequality itself. Rather than the traditional health promotion focus on the amelioration of the health effects of poverty, some authors are suggesting a broader focus on the structure of society and the actions of the advantaged in perpetuating inequalities (e.g., Scambler, 2002; Chapman and Berggren, 2005; Stephens, 2008). Murray and Campbell (2003) have called upon health psychologists to develop 'actionable under-standings' of the relationships and structures underlying health inequalities. Mabala (2006) has made a very clear case for such actionable understandings. He shows that HIV/AIDS in urban Africa flourishes in situations of poverty and severe inequity, with young women and girls particularly vulnerable to this situation. He points to the need to address the underlying causes of this inequality including the effects of globalization: debt burdens, trade inequities and priorities of aid donors.

Values and ethical issues in choosing models for practice

Which models are chosen for implementation will depend upon the health promoter's own values and understandings of the basis of health. These fundamental values will influence the health promoters' choice to draw on social, humanist or positivist scientific theories to explain health and to choose particular models of health promotion practice. Furthermore, these models produce particular situations which raise their own ethical issues.

Health promotion as a moral endeavour

Seedhouse (1997) sees health promotion as unequivocally a moral endeavour. From this perspective he considers ethical issues in general health promotion practice by making two sets of distinctions: first, between health promotion aimed at a defined individual or group or at the population; second, between health promotion on request or health promotion without the recipients asking for it. These two distinctions lead to four alternatives:

A. Health promotion to improve public health in accordance with the clear wishes of the public.
B. Health promotion on request of a specifically defined individual or group.
C. Health promotion to improve the health of a specific individual or group without that group requesting it.
D. Health promotion to improve the general public health without the expressed consent of the general public or at the request of a minority interest group

(p. 170)

Seedhouse considers that for A and B a health promoter will be able to review the ethical requirements for practice (such as reflection on her own prejudices, qualifications to provide information, assessment of evidence or costs for others) and proceed with few qualms. Each case gets slightly more complex and for C there are an additional set of aspects to consider (such as the intrusiveness of the intervention, the needs of the recipients, and the moral dimensions of the issue). For D, large scale interventions for which it is difficult to gain everybody's consent, there are all the ethical issues of the first three, plus an absolute requirement for 'having, demonstrating, explaining and abiding by a defensible, explicit theory of intervention for health' (p. 172).

The values of health promotion practice

From a community perspective, Guttman (2000) assesses the different ways in which participants may be involved in health promotion intervention and their ethical implications. Guttman sees community involvement as a value in itself, and describes four models of intervention differentiating between whether involvement is a goal or a strategy or both:

A. Service: Community involvement is low as a goal and strategy (e.g. health services such as screening for risk factors).
B. Collaboration: Community involvement low as a goal but high as a strategy (e.g. interventions that rely on community based organisa-tions to implement the health objectives).
C. Augmentation: Community involvement is high as a goal but low as a strategy (e.g. interventions that emphasise involvement but do not enhance capacities of community members).
D. Mobilization: Community involvement is high as both goal and strategy (e.g. helps facilitate involvement of community based groups and individuals to determine the issues and how to address them)

(p. 143)

Guttman provides a useful illustration of the differences between two interventions with the same ostensible goal: to increase child immunization rates in a low income population. The first intervention employs com-munity residents as peer educators to disseminate messages about parental responsibility for children's immunization. The second employs community members who decide to focus on the role and ability of parents to influence the allocation of health care resources in their community. The use of Guttman's typology assists us to compare such situations and consider how the community resources are deployed, who is in control and what ethical issues may be involved. Taking Guttman's approach means that principles such as participation, empowerment and capacity building are seen as values with their successful implementation considered in terms of ethical issues and dilemmas.

Guttman provides a detailed analysis of the values and ethical issues raised by the four scenarios. Briefly, when community involvement as a goal is emphasized the values are autonomy, participation, empowerment and self-determination. Strategies should enable people to gain mastery and facilitate changes. The ethical issues arise around the actual practice of these goals and strategies in terms of the political functioning of communities and who is represented and who actually has control. Related ethical issues arise when community members suggest problems or solutions that will not be efficacious according to the knowledge or values of the health professionals. An example of such a dilemma comes from Campbell's (2003) evaluation of an AIDS prevention programme in South Africa. The participatory programme involved the local administrative committee and peer educators. Both of these groups used coercion and beatings to force women to attend education meetings or to punish them for not using condoms. Although these methods were part of the local culture at the time, it was difficult for the outside programme coordinators to condone these methods.

When community involvement as a strategy is emphasized, the values are those of hierarchy, expertise and possibly paternalism. These values are most apparent in the service (A) model in which the health promotion goal is well defined and the lead organization controls decisions and resources. The ethical issues that arise in these situations are the use of limited community resources for outside goals, collaborations which develop 'vertical communities' serving as a mechanism to deploy outside power, non-representation of the community (those who participate in such organizations tend to be from more privileged groups), and blame falling on the community itself for any failures.

Political implications of choosing strategies

A number of authors, particularly those concerned with inequalities in health and social justice, are pointing to the very negative effects of choosing certain dominant approaches to health promotion. Barnes (2007, p. 531) describes the dominance of behavioural change and individually focused interventions in developing countries. He suggests that framing interventions within 'a mainstream environmental health science paradigm' works on several levels to:

◆ Set up an 'expert' model of science.
◆ Shut out other development options.
◆ Perpetuate sexist representations of African women.
◆ Allow decision makers to ignore the key sociopolitical determinants of health such as poverty and inequality.

Barnes provides an example of the different possibilities of approaching health issues in impoverished areas. In a resource poor town in South Africa, the department of health responded to an outbreak of typhoid by setting up temporary health care facilities, temporary clean water points for the residents, and a behavioural campaign to promote disposal of waste and hand washing. The residents of the town 'mobilised in protest'. They saw the outbreak as lack of services such as clean water, flush sanitation and healthcare facilities to impoverished areas. 'The residents used an equity/human rights perspective . . . The State used an environmental health science paradigm focussing on specific disease . . .' (p. 532).

Mabala (2006) also points to the effects of particular perspectives that determine prevention methods on the HIV/AIDS campaigns in Africa. According to Mabala, the dominance of a moralist perspective, in which individual behaviour is seen as the cause, is hindering the progress of

HIV/AIDS prevention and directly leading to neglect of the powerful evidence for the role of poverty, inequality and lack of social cohesion. In particular, Mabala suggests that adolescent girls and young women are bearing the brunt of this neglect. He argues that behavioural change interventions cannot reach these women who are nevertheless the most vulnerable to the disease. Only attention to their social and economic circumstances including policies that provide for protection and social participation for these girls and young women, and attention to the broader underlying causes will help prevent the spread of disease. While arguing for social and political change Mabala is also pointing to the damaging and oppositional effects of a powerful and dominant perspective, which he sees as based in an alternative set of values.

Prilleltensky and Prillelltensky (2003) used a critical psychology framework to review the whole field of health psychology on the basis of assumptions, values and practice. These authors suggest that the most promising way to promote health is to work with whole communities proactively (rather than working with those affected or at risk of illness). In doing so, power issues and justice are of paramount importance in considering ethical issues. Bolam and Chamberlain (2003) agree with these arguments and add that reflexivity must take a central place in health practice. A reflexive approach is aimed toward making apparent the theoretical, moral and political assumptions and the value laden choices of any approach to health promotion.

Summary

In this chapter, we moved from considering ways of understanding health from a social perspective, to understandings of how we can work toward improving the health of people in communities and populations. To continue on from the sections on theory and research methodology, this chapter overviewed theoretical approaches to health promotion intervention itself. The range of different theoretical approaches to health promotion intervention were described under the very broadly descriptive categories of, 'ecological' models, 'social determinants' models, and 'local and cultural' models, as well as some approaches to health promotion messages broadcast through the media and some of the different ways in which the broader structural and political issues in health have been addressed.

These descriptions of a range of the theoretical models that are presently in use should not be taken as a comprehensive overview. Rather, these examples are offered as illustrations of the sorts of models that are available with some examples of their application and some critiques and problems that have been encountered using each approach. I hope that the reader will take these examples as an indication of the variety of approaches to the practice of health promotion from a social and environmental perspective, and an invitation to pursue areas of interest in more depth. In addition, I hope that the discussion of values underlying the choice of particular theoretical approaches, and of the ethical issues involved in making these choices will encourage reflection on our own values and choices of action.

The next chapter will provide some more detailed examples of the application of different models of community-based health promotion as an opportunity to make some comparisons and consider some of the issues around health promotion practice in more depth.

Further reading

1 For those who are interested in the use of social cognitive models in health promotion work, this book draws on work from several contributors to provide examples of the application of these models. The final chapter addresses the difficulties of using these theories to design interventions:

Rutter, D. and Quine, L. (eds) (2002) *Changing Health Behaviour*. Buckingham: Open University Press.

2 For those who are interested in the application of the social capital concept, this paper provides an excellent review of the use of social capital in health promotion and many of the issues raised by the application of popular concepts:

Hawe, P. and Shiell, A. (2000) Social capital and health promotion: a review, *Social Science & Medicine*, 51(6), 871–85.

3 For those interested in PAR, the first paper provides a very considered and systematic overview of the ideological and ethical issues in PAR approaches to community health programmes. Written to assist reviewers, it also provides a clear set of guidelines for practitioners to consider. The second paper considers ethical issues in the use of PAR in a particular context; and the third paper provides a further example of the recent use of PAR with specific populations:

Khanlou, N. and Peter, E. (2005) Participatory action research: considerations for ethical review, *Social Science & Medicine*, 60, 2333–40.

Ellis, B.H., Kia-Keating, M., Yusuf, S.A., Lincoln, A. and Nur, A. (2007) Ethical research in refugee communities and the use of community participartory methods, *Transcultural Psychiatry*, 44, 459–81.

Liu, M., Gao, R. and Pusari, N. (2006) Using participatory action research to provide health promotion for disadvantaged elders in Shaanxi Province, China, *Public Health Nursing*, 23(4), 332–8.

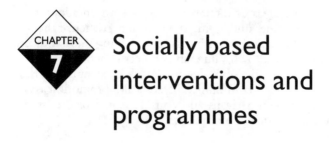

Socially based interventions and programmes

Introduction

This chapter focuses on some specific examples of social and community approaches to health promotion. These examples have been chosen to indicate the wide range of health issues; diversity in community health promotion practice; different theoretical approaches to understanding the issue and its determinants; and different levels and models from which the determinants may be addressed. In considering the examples that are described below we need to bring our critical faculties to bear and ask questions such as, why these issues, why this conceptualization of the issues and why this approach? Some more detailed questions are posed at the end of this chapter to aid reflection.

The examples of socially based interventions described below are available in the literature for more detailed consideration. Here, they are briefly outlined in terms of:

1 The evidence for the issue that is the basis for intervention, and the theories or explanations of this health issue.
2 The objectives of the intervention programme.
3 The theories of health promotion that are used as models for the intervention.
4 The practical implementation of the objectives.

Evaluation of the interventions will also be mentioned if appropriate, although this important aspect of any intervention will be developed in the next chapter.

The issues themselves provide very diverse objectives for intervention. First, we will consider seven different interventions that were targeted to two specific medically defined health issues: chronic illnesses such as diabetes and HIV/AIDS. Second, we will consider four examples of interventions in particular communities which take a broader approach to health.

Interventions targeted to medical issues: chronic illness prevention and care

Commumity intervention in Finland based on a social cognitive model

Type 2 diabetes mellitus is seen as a serious costly disease in most of the Western world. Prevention, targeted at diet and exercise as underlying causes, is the preferred medical approach, which also recognizes that successful interventions in some societies may not work in others because social, economic and cultural forces influence diet and exercise (Diabetes Prevention Program Research Group, 2002).

In line with these understandings, Uutela et al. (2004) describe a community programme for type 2 diabetes prevention that has been implemented by Finnish primary health care services. All information about this programme is from that paper. The programme recruited participants through primary health care centres or public health nurse visits in one district. People determined to be at risk for developing type 2 diabetes (through a questionnaire based on epidemiological studies of risk factors) were invited to participate in group education sessions (12 to a group, with 40 groups operating in the district in 2003).

Evidence and theoretical basis for understanding diabetes as a health issue

This programme is part of a broader health promotion project based in one district which was found to have higher than average rates of mortality. To provide a rationale for diabetes prevention as a specific target, the authors cited statistics that show diabetes is a growing public health problem in Finland with increases of incidence predicted. They provided medical explanations of how diabetes is understood as the result of a high fat, low fibre diet and sedentary lifestyle. They also describe evidence to show that they cannot simply draw on previous successful programmes in Finland. As the social context has changed, people's understandings of diet have shifted and diets have generally improved, although activity has meanwhile decreased so that obesity remains an underlying issue.

Objectives

According to medical theory and evidence, the causes of obesity are located in individual health related behaviours. Therefore, one of the main aims was to develop a cost effective lifestyle change programme for use in primary health care. The aim of the intervention was that participants would modify their diet and exercise to achieve very specific goals (Uutela et al., 2004, p. 79):

1 No more that 30 percent of total energy from fat.
2 No more than 10 percent of total energy from saturated fats.

3 At least 15g/1000 kcal of fibre.
4 At least 30 min./day moderate intensity physical activity.
5 At least 5 percent reduction in body weight.

Theoretical model for intervention

To understand the behaviour change participants must make to achieve these goals, Uutela and colleagues drew on the health action process approach (HAPA). This is a social cognitive model of behaviour change that begins with an account of processes of intention formation, but additionally includes understandings of planning and action. To explain the cognitions that influence actual behaviour the model draws on theories of self-efficacy and self-regulation (see Schwarzer, 2008, for a full account of this model). The determinants of exercise and dietary behaviour change specified by the HAPA model (2004, p. 79) were that the participants should:

♦ Acknowledge that they are at risk for type 2 diabetes.
♦ Learn that the disease can be prevented by certain lifestyle changes.
♦ Gain confidence in their ability to make the changes.
♦ Make a decision to make the changes.
♦ Plan where, when and how to make the changes.

Implementation

The programme included six two-hour sessions facilitated by trained health care professionals. The facilitator enabled and moderated discussions, gave homework assignments and strengthened the role of the group so that participants can learn from each other (p. 80). The sessions drew on existing health education materials (such as advice about diet or exercise schedules) with additional materials which draw on the HAPA model. Specific sessions were designed to target the steps specified by the HAPA model (intention formations; planning and action):

♦ *Sessions 1 and 2 – intention formation.* The cognitions that influence intentions are risk perception (I'm at risk for diabetes); outcome expectation (lifestyle changes reduce the risk); and self-efficacy (I can make a change). Information and guided discussion activities addressed these cognitions.
♦ *Sessions 3 and 4 – planning for exercise and diet change.* Goals were individually tailored to fit with the participants' normal routines and to be achievable.
♦ *Sessions 5 and 6 – action phase.* Refining plans and moving towards goals was the emphasis, taking into account the effects of environmental factors on self-efficacy.

Conclusions

The strength of this programme is the clarity and coherence of conceptualization from evidence to practice. The programme is very clearly based in the context of epidemiological evidence, medical theories of the causes of illness, and a social cognitive model of health related behaviour and behaviour change. Evaluation of the constructs and outcomes specified by these goals is planned but no results available yet.

Community intervention in the US based on a participatory model

In the 1970s WHO placed community participation at the forefront of their strategy to achieve health for all. This was seen as a shift from the medical model of care (Zakus and Lysack, 1998) and the Ottawa Charter stressed the role of community action in deciding on the causes and solutions of health issues. Resulting models of participation have been implemented at different levels of community participation. A community needs assessment and community walking intervention in one town in Washington County, in the US, is an example of a community and university partnership. Here community members are consulted at every step of the way about the issues, while the university researchers bring outside knowledge about the community's health problems as well as some broader theoretical models of the causes of those problems.

Evidence and theoretical basis for understanding the health issue

Ndirangu et al. (2007) describe a needs assessment project using the comprehensive participatory planning and evaluation model (CPPE). A university and government agency consortium first identified the Lower Mississippi Delta region as an area with high rates of chronic disease such as diabetes, and also high fat and low fibre diets in the population. For one arm of the project, the consortium chose Hollandale, a community with low income and high risk factors such as higher unemployment and poverty. Citizens of Hollandale and academics formed a partnership to address the identified health and nutrition concerns.

Objectives

Thirty community and university representatives were invited to two all-day CPPE workshops (Zoellner et al., 2007). The objectives were to:

1 Identify key problems and issues contributing to nutrition and health status.
2 Identify skill targets and resource factors associated with the problems.
3 Identify objectives and activities to address key problems.

The three foremost problems identified were lack of physical activity, eating unhealthy food and lack of nutrition knowledge. The workshop participants developed causal models of these problems, which were used to identify the objectives and activities to address the causes. Zoellner et al. (2007) describe a community walking intervention that was developed in response to the physical activity problem identified in this process.

Theoretical model for intervention

The intervention is based on community participatory research (CBPR) methodology to link community members with academic and government partners. This collaboration is seen as facilitating the joint identification of health problems and collaborative development and implementation of intervention strategies. In developing the intervention the researchers drew on the causal model of physical activity developed by the CPPE. This model included environmental issues such as lack of facilities and individual factors such as motivation, knowledge, and family constraints (see Ndirangu et al., 2007).

In addition they applied two theoretical frameworks to understand exercise adoption activity (Zoellner et al., 2007). Social support which has been established in the literature as a predictor of exercise and associated with the adoption of exercise suggested the importance of social aspects of exercise. The transtheoretical model (TTM) of behaviour change was also drawn on to suggest the importance of three cognitions: stage of change (readiness to exercise); self-efficacy (confidence in one's ability to exercise); and decisional balance (assessment of the benefits and costs of exercise).

Implementation

In response to the identification of environmental causes, the Hollandale research partnership, city and businesses collaborated to build a walking trail. The research group was then encouraged to initiate an intervention to promote use of the trail.

The details of the walking promotion intervention were based on other examples of community-based approaches in the literature. The six-month intervention employed walking teams led by supportive coaches. The coaches were community members nominated by the research group. They were trained across three sessions to recruit participants, and led their walking team by contacting them to encourage goal setting and walking and to collect weekly walking logs. Group walking was encouraged but not required.

Five one-hour education sessions on topics such as nutrition and healthy body mass index were delivered to all participants with a final celebration session. At each session coaches received a report on their team's activity.

Incentives such as water bottles and recipe boxes were given at group meetings. Coaches received six $25 payments for returning records and assisting.

Forty coaches were nominated and eight participated by leading a total of 88 members. These numbers declined to 58 at the final data collection. Younger members were most likely to drop out.

Conclusion

Many of the theoretical constructs of behaviour change were apparently applied to the evaluation measures rather than to the design of the intervention itself. The results of measurements taken at enrolment, three months and six months showed improvement for participants in biological measures such as waist circumference and blood pressure, although not in BMI or overall net increase in walking. There were no significant changes in the psychosocial variables of social support or those specified by the TTM.

Community intervention in Canada based on a participatory model

Potvin et al. (2003) justify the use of a participatory community approach to diabetes prevention through principles of social justice and equity in health. They draw on the WHO definition of health promotion as enabling people and communities to control health, and also recent commentaries and research, which argue that the active participation of citizens in public health programmes can reduce inequalities and promote social justice. In addition they suggest that traditional approaches to health promotion that are based on expert knowledge and detailed advance planning may be especially unhelpful in community programmes, and may not address the needs of Aboriginal communities.

Evidence and theoretical basis for understanding the health issue

Macauley et al. (1997) describe a community-based prevention programme for type 2 diabetes in an indigenous community in Canada. First they provide evidence to show that diabetes is a recent and growing health threat to indigenous populations and why. They also provide evidence for obesity as the predominant risk factor for diabetes, and for physical inactivity and dietary factors as predictors of obesity in these populations. The Mohawk community of Kahnawake chosen for this intervention also had a rate of adult incidence of type 2 diabetes that was twice the rate of the general population.

These authors go on to provide a strong rationale for the target group. The intervention was youth centred on the basis of evidence for intergenerational risk; increasing early incidence; and that behaviours and overweight continue from youth to adulthood unless changed. Also they proposed that school children are a captive audience ready to learn. As a community centred intervention, the programme included the whole population on the basis of findings showing that a general population approach is more effective than screening and targeting at risk groups (p. 788).

Objectives

Thus, the programme has a long-term goal of decreasing future occurrence of type 2 diabetes. Short-term goals were to reduce the prevalence of obesity, high calorie diets and physical inactivity among Kahawake children of 6–12 years; and specifically to increase the proportion of children who have a balanced diet and regular activity.

Theoretical model for intervention

The model for intervention combined several theoretical elements:

1 A participatory approach of community consultation and inclusion.
2 The Ottawa Charter for Health Promotion was used to identify specific axes of capacity building: developing personal skills; strengthening community action; creating supportive environments; building healthy public policy; and re-orienting health services.
3 Social learning theory, in particular the constructs of self-efficacy (behavioural change effected through mastery); modelling (of behaviours by role models); and self-management (internal gratification).
4 The precede–proceed model which identifies predisposing (children's knowledge and skills); reinforcing (support of teachers and family); and enabling (availability of healthy foods and opportunities for activity) factors.
5 An overriding principle was to incorporate traditional learning styles of indigenous children.

Implementation

The programme was based on principles of participation at every level. Community members had requested an intervention when they were shown local diabetes statistics. A community advisory board was created with 40 members from many sectors. The board advised on intervention objectives, activities, culture, traditions and current concerns. Board members also become role models. Two full-time Mohawk staff members coordinated the intervention and Mohawk school teachers additionally provided local expertise. The programme also made extensive use of the media to inform and involve the public, and supported existing community groups and events such as the youth recreation centre, health and harvest fairs, and sports competitions.

Over three years, a new health education programme was introduced into the elementary schools and this was supported by 63 different activities for the children, teachers, families and community. These activities drew upon principles specified by the intervention models.

The models and principles of health promotion were integrated throughout the education programme and many community activities. For example, the education programme in schools drew on the social learning theory constructs and traditional learning styles to develop personal skills specified by the Ottawa Charter. In addition the modelling aspect of social learning theory was developed through family activities in the community to show children healthy lifestyles. Teacher training for the health education programme, healthy classroom activities and presentations about healthy eating to community organizations were developed to strengthen the predisposing factors suggested by the precede–proceed model. To develop the enabling factors of this model, the programme successfully lobbied the local education system for active reinforcement of the school nutrition policy, and school canteens now offer only healthy foods. Teachers and schools were also encouraged to add extra physical education classes each week (see Macauley et al., 1997 for a detailed overview).

Conclusions

Potvin et al. (2003) have evaluated this programme to develop four principles that should be the basic components of participatory interventions which are negotiated in an ongoing process. They suggest:

1 The integration of community people and researchers at every phase.
2 The structural and functional integration of evaluation and research.
3 Having a flexible agenda responsive to demands from the environment.
4 A project that creates learning opportunities for all involved.

A diabetes self-care intervention in England based on a narrative approach

For those who have developed type 2 diabetes a great deal of intervention work at clinical and community levels is conducted to support the self-care that is required to manage this chronic illness. Training in how to self-manage diabetes has long been considered an important part of clinical management (Norris et al., 2001). The aim of training is to develop knowledge, attitudes, self-care skills including glycemic control, changes in important lifestyle behaviours such as diet and exercise, and coping skills. Such interventions are usually based on psychological approaches to individual change and a review has shown that they are generally effective in the short-term (Norris et al., 2001). These reviewers also concluded that educational interventions involving patient collaboration are more effective, and that few studies have examined health care utilization as an issue.

Collaboration and utilization may be the very issues that result in the poor diabetes outcomes for some harder to reach groups such as ethnic minorities.

Evidence and theoretical basis for understanding the health issue

Greenhalgh et al. (2005a) present evidence showing that the outcomes of diabetes are often worse for members of different ethnic groups in the UK. In particular the rates of incidence of diabetes and illness from complications for ethnic Asian people are higher than for white people. The complex reasons include socioeconomic deprivation, genetic risk, discrimination and racism, exercise and food choices, communication, and access to services (Greenhalgh et al., 2005b). Thus, members of these more vulnerable groups are much less likely to attend lifestyle interventions as they are isolated from mainstream services and often speak little English. These authors suggest that an anthropological perspective to diabetes self-management interventions is useful in this context. This approach takes into account the shared values and meanings of different behaviours for members of different cultures who may be excluded from main stream services.

Objectives

The aim was to develop diabetes support and education for minority ethnic groups. An action research framework (see Greenhalgh et al., 2005b) was used to collect data systematically and successively throughout the project to evaluate progress and develop new goals at each step. For example, after training the advocates, it became clear that organizational support was an essential part of the programme. Many of the advocates were confident and committed after training but had little power to implement the sessions in their own organizations and required extra support. The goals for each stage became:

1 Map the extent of diabetes and level of diabetes care in the locality and develop partnerships with key stakeholders and other local initiatives.
2 Train a group of bilingual health advocates (BHAs) to run support and education groups.
3 Support the BHAs to pilot diabetes groups for clients in health care sites.
4 Set up and sustain BHA led education and support groups for diabetes service users.

Theoretical model for intervention

At the heart of these objectives is the design of the education groups and training for the BHAs. For this aspect of the complex intervention, a narrative approach was chosen. The authors' previous research had shown that positive behaviour changes (such as giving up smoking) in British Bangladeshis was often attributed to a story told in an informal setting by another Bangladeshi. Drawing upon narrative theory and clinical application Greenhalgh et al. (2005b) described why narratives are applicable to health education:

♦ Stories are a natural and universal form of communication.
♦ Stories create engagement through metaphor, rich imagery, suspense and other literary devices.
♦ Stories are sense-making devices – i.e., they allow people to make sense of events and actions and link them to past experience.
♦ Stories embrace complexity. They can capture all the elements of a problem.
♦ Stories offer insights into what might (could or should) have been, and hence consider different options and their likely endings.
♦ Stories have an ethical dimension, and hence motivate the learner.
♦ Stories occur in both formal and informal space. Hence, story-based learning can occur from a very wide range of sources.
♦ Stories are performative. They focus attention on actions (and inactions) and provide lessons for how actions could change in future situations.

Implementation

The first training set was restricted to 13 Bangladeshi female advocates. Subsequently, Gujarati, Persian, Somalian, Turkish, Arabic and Chinese speakers of both sexes were included in courses.

Management in the health care centres were engaged to provide organizational support for the programme.

Different advocate led user groups developed their own format and identity, which was sometimes quite different to the anticipated format. For example, in one group a weekly 'diabetes storytelling group' grew from eight to 42 regular attenders in 18 months. Participants were not willing to be organized by the research team, but used them as a resource to answer questions or comment on a story. 'To a visitor the group would have seemed chaotic with multiple conversations co-occurring at once and women wandering around the room, coming and going as they pleased, and often bringing friends or grandchildren with them' (Greenhalgh et al., 2005a, p. 632).

Conclusions

The authors conclude that this approach was successful in engaging these hard to reach groups of service users with good initial results. The complex intervention will be tested in formal trials.

Interventions targeted to medical issues – HIV/AIDS prevention

Critics of the dominant individual behaviour change approach to the HIV/
AIDS epidemic like Richard Mabala (2006), point to the evidence strongly
demonstrating that AIDS flourishes in situations of poverty and inequity.
In many developing countries, such as India, South Africa or Cambodia, the
low status of women is a key social determinant of health (Assai et al., 2006),
and this makes women especially vulnerable to HIV infection. Farmer
(Lubek, 2003) has argued for a more systemic and critical perspective that
does not accept simple causality explanations. Increasing numbers of commentators are similarly calling for interventions that include the evidence
for roles of complex relationships between gender, inequality, poverty
and the patterns of distribution of HIV. Here, three interventions that
have attempted community and multilevel approaches to these issues are
introduced.

A social psychological approach to participatory interventions to prevent AIDS in South Africa

In *Letting Them Die: Why HIV/Intervention Programmes Fail* Catherine
Campbell has used the evaluation of a 'gold-standard' HIV/AIDS intervention project (Gibbs, 2007) to develop a social psychological theory of community participation. As part of this complex evaluation (which will be
revisited in Chapter 8) she describes the basis of a participatory HIV/AIDS
prevention project, which will be outlined here based on the 2003 book.
The programme was based in a town in South Africa which is typical of
the sort of environment in which the current epidemic has thrived: it has
100,000 permanent residents, 70,000 migrants who work in the mines,
and 2000 commercial sex workers.

Evidence and theoretical basis for understanding the health issue

Campbell (2003) cites evidence to show that on many levels there is a crisis
in sub-Saharan Africa and the fight against HIV/AIDS is one of the biggest
challenges for this region and the world. Although there are myriad issues
concerning those with the disease, prevention remains an important goal.

In considering prevention activities Campbell introduces a social psychology approach to sexuality that is located at the community level. According to Campbell, local community is where our well demonstrated but
presently quite separate understandings of individual motivations and perceptions, and of the effects of structural factors such as poverty, gender
inequalities and capitalism, meet. 'Local communities often form the contexts within which people negotiate their social and sexual lives and
identities' (p.3). The interaction between individual behaviour and structural
factors occurs in this context because as community social mores shape

people's needs and behaviours, so the broader social and economic factors shape those communities.

Thus, while Campbell draws on evidence that STIs increase risk of HIV/AIDS, she notes that behaviour that apparently ignores these risks is not due to ignorance. People in these communities are well aware of the high death rate and the causes of the epidemic. Information and motivation is not sufficient to ensure behavioural change. It is the mores of a person's social group and the structure of social interactions that must be addressed.

Objectives

On the basis of these understandings, the project was designed to address the medical and social issues of the HIV/AIDS epidemic in the town with three broad aims:

1 STI control by addressing social norms of sexual behaviour and relationships.
2 To reach particular at-risk social groups (not individuals).
3 To engage the broader community (private and public sector, and civil society) whose actions affect these groups.

Theoretical model for intervention

The framework for the intervention drew on three theoretical explanations:

1 Social psychological understandings of sexuality as socially constructed.
2 The notion of a 'health enabling community', which recognizes that broader contextual factors support the performance of health related behaviours such as condom use. Past efforts to combat HIV/AIDS have failed because they have relied on biomedical and behavioural interventions to target individuals. The development of a 'health enabling community' promotes the supportive social processes that empower people to protect themselves.
3 A participatory framework which is aimed at encouraging local people to collectively take ownership of the problem and to engage in collective action to improve sexual health. These participants included:
    ♦ the local at-risk community groups;
    ♦ stakeholders from the broader community as partners.

Implementation

The aims were addressed within this framework through local multistakeholder collaborative project management of a community led peer education and condom distribution programme.

The project was initiated by a group of black African residents of a township in a gold mining region in South Africa. The group included teachers, social workers, youth leaders, traditional healers and mine officials all concerned about HIV/AIDS. They were introduced to academics interested in research in AIDS prevention work. After lengthy negotiations, the project's stakeholder group was formed including the initiating group, mine management, trade unions, provincial and national government, and several researchers and international funding agencies. The stakeholders set up an NGO which employed three local full-time workers and a coordinator based in Johannesburg.

For the purpose of the project, the community was defined as all those living in the geographical area of the town, which includes a small town centre, a black township at a distance and miners' hostels just out of town. Sex workers live in squatter settlements outside the mines. These arrangements are the immediate legacy of the apartheid system. There is a great deal of poverty and crime in the township, with poor educational facilities and high unemployment. Three key social groups in the town who were highlighted as being at risk for HIV/AIDS were the mine workers, sex workers and the town's youth. At the project's outset, 69 percent of the sex workers, 22 percent of the miners, and 8 percent of the town's 15-year-old girls were HIV-positive.

Community led peer education was initiated in these three groups. The peer education programme was designed to train volunteer members of each community to motivate their peers to change the collective social constructions of sexuality that endangered their health. The different economic, social and political needs of these groups were taken into account. Overall, the aim was not to *persuade* people to change their behaviour but to 'turn their attention to the possibility of creating circumstances that *enable* behaviour change' (p. 35; emphasis in original).

Conclusion

Campbell concludes that our understanding of what creates a 'health enabling community' is in its infancy. Evaluation of this programme has shown that community programmes to prevent HIV infection and AIDS must work for change on many levels at once. First, they must take into account the relationships *between* separate groups and not just within them. Especially where the social and economic forces between groups (such as sex workers and miners) are those that increase their shared risk of HIV infection. This means that all members of the relevant community must have a meaningful role in designing and executing the project since they have the fullest understanding of local conditions and constraints. Second, programmes must take into account and address the power imbalances that allow some 'stakeholders' to withhold information and otherwise actively counter community efforts. Thus, the fight against HIV/AIDS must be a multilayered effort that includes consideration of the role of, not just grass roots community groups but also many others with competing interests including donors, experts, political leaders and business groups.

A multilevel participatory approach to AIDS prevention in Cambodia

Siem Reap Citizens for Health, Educational and Social Issues (SiRCHESI) is a Cambodian non-governmental organization confronting an HIV/AIDS epidemic in Siem Reap, the town situated next to Cambodia's major tourist attraction, the Angkor Wat temple complex.

Evidence and theoretical basis for understanding the health issue

In Siem Reap, which has a population of 140,000, 10,000 persons were sero-positive in 2006 (see www.angkorwatngo.com). Local research has shown that there are up to 40,000 sex tourists in a year. These visitors often drink heavily and do not use condoms with the brothel-based sex workers (about 44 percent HIV-positive) and beer promotion women (about 15–33 percent HIV-positive) who, underpaid by international beer companies and coerced to overdrink nightly with their customers, some-times exchange unprotected sex for money. Local men, single and married, also have sex with these women, without a condom, about 20 percent of the time. Fewer than 10 percent of the married men use condoms and 15 percent of their wives tested HIV-positive in 2001. HIV is also being transferred to newborns. With rates of HIV seropositivity between 15 and 44 percent for samples of female sex workers, the HIV+ rate for pregnant women rose from 5 percent in 2000 to 11 percent in 2001 (Lubek et al., 2003).

Thus, the HIV/AIDS epidemic is understood as being related to inconsistent condom use within a social context of sexual tourism, poverty and exploitation of workers, compounded by workplace health/safety risks, especially to women (violence, alcohol overuse, sexual exploitation and trafficking).

Objectives

The aims of the project are to develop a multisector capacity building research and health intervention programme to:

1 Reduce the spread of sexually transmitted infections in Siem Reap.
2 Address inequalities in literacy, employment, poverty and risk of dying from HIV/AIDS (Lubek et al., 2003).

These aims have generated specific objectives at different levels:

1 Individual behavioural change to 100 percent condom use for those at risk.

2 Social development including provision of peer support, literacy education, and employment opportunities.
3 Changes in local employment conditions.
4 The involvement of globalized businesses.

Theoretical model for intervention

The model of participatory action research, originally proposed by Kurt
Lewin as 'action research' has guided this project since 2000. This model
begins with community contact prior to problem definition, and as
methods and data collection develop, collective interpretation of results to
determine what further action should be taken, or cycling back to redefine
the problem and the research process. Thus, community participation and
feedback have co-determined the goals and methods (Lubek et al., 2006).

Implementation

This model means that research and intervention methods are intertwined
in the cycles of feedback, action, consultation and research. Here the activities of what is actually a complex multisectoral programme will be outlined
according to spheres of action:

1 *Research*. The programme supports ongoing enquiry into the social and
  medical situation with results fed back directly to local groups.
      Initially interviews were conducted to enquire into citizens' experi-
  ences during the genocide period, their current lifestyle, including risk
  taking and sexual activity, and their views of the future in Cambodia.
  After hearing a summary of the results of these interviews, the participants formed a grass roots social action group to address the social, educational and medical needs highlighted. SiRCHESI was then formally
  established to conduct ongoing research and development of educational
  and medical interventions (Lubek et al., 2002).
      For example, systematic behavioural surveying of groups at risk since
  2001 (sex workers, 'beer promotion women', local men, married women)
  allows SiRCHESI and the Department of Health to continuously monitor sexual practices related to HIV/AIDS risk. Strategies to counter risky
  behaviours are then integrated into community peer educator workshops. New directions in prevention (e.g., workshops for men, for young
  persons or for couples) have arisen from this 'feedback loop' (Kros et al.,
  2004).
2 *Individual and community level*. Based on feedback from research, a pyra-
  midal 'peer educator' training programme was initiated and a peer educational intervention project designed to provide strategies for behaviour
  change to groups of women highlighted as at risk for HIV/AIDS.
  Educational materials successfully used in Singapore and Malaysia were

translated into Khmer and first tested in focus groups for cultural appropriateness (Lubek et al., 2003).

Social behaviour change strategies and negotiation techniques were taught to peer educator trainers in target groups: beer promotion women, married men, pregnant women and young souvenir vendors facing predatory sex tourists. These outreach activities have expanded from 25 beer promoters and 25 married women in 2002, to over 4000 in 2006, including men's groups (Liu and Ng, 2007).

Community meetings have been held to create an all-in-one clinic for HIV/AIDS prevention, education, acute care, diagnosis, treatment, long-term care and follow-up. This centre coordinates all activities and explores broader institutional cooperation with other NGOs, medical practitioners, hospitals, international funding sources, government agencies, and the local and international business sector (Lubek et al., 2002).

3 *Community and local institutional level.* SiRCHESI works with other NGOs, hospitals, agencies and government organizations to strengthen the public health sector, partnering with the Provincial AIDS Office and the provincial department of health.

In 2006–08, SiRCHESI partnered with three Siem Reap hotels in a hotel apprenticeship programme to remove women from risky beer selling jobs. The programme provides education in English language, Khmer reading, health and life skills. For eight months apprentices complete mentored shifts at the hotels and then receive 16-month contracts, with fair wages paid throughout.

New Cambodian health and safety legislation for women has been promoted and there are moves to form solidarity groups of beer promoters (Lubek et al., 2006).

4 *International activism.* An international group has worked to raise financial support, and mobilize public and corporate support for increased efforts to confront the HIV/AIDS epidemic in Cambodia (Lubek et al., 2004).

Globalized beer companies have been challenged to contribute proactively to the campaign against the spread of HIV/AIDS in several ways. Shareholders, trade unions and pension plan managers have been encouraged to take action to improve their company's workplace policies in Cambodia (Lubek et al., 2003; Lubek et al., 2004).

Several website information campaigns, concerning the ethical and fair-trade practices of international beer companies (e.g., www.angkorwatngo. com, www.beergirls.org and www.fairtradebeer.com) have been developed in international locations.

The international partners publish press reports (see www. angkorwatngo. com) to publicize the broader social and industrial issues. Academics write to medical journals (Van Merode et al., 2006), present papers at conferences (Lubek et al., 2005), and present seminars and talks around the world (Liu and Ng, 2007), to highlight the industrial issues, and the responsibility of beer companies to stop the unfair practices which have serious health effects for workers.

Conclusion

Data from behavioural health surveys (2001–06) and continuous serological testing in Siem Reap, indicate that HIV prevalence rates may be decreasing. The broader issues, like workplace overdrinking, violence, harassment, sexual exploitation and trafficking, need additional attention from researchers/practitioners (Lubek et al., 2006).

A participatory AIDS prevention project among sex workers in India

The Sonagachi Project is a longstanding, community-based intervention that has developed successfully across time (Mukherjea, 2006). It was founded in Calcutta in 1991 as the Sexually Transmitted Diseases/HIV Intervention Project by the All India Institute of Hygiene and Public Health. It is now run by the Durbar Mahila Samanwaya Committee (DMSC), a 6000 strong sex workers' body in West Bengal.

Evidence and theoretical basis for understanding the health issue

In describing the development of this programme, Jana et al., (2004) describe AIDS as an important health threat to India and to Indian sex workers in particular. They also provide evidence to support the role of community level and structural factors, rather than individual behaviour, in the epidemiology of HIV/AIDS internationally. Sex workers are vulnerable to HIV transmission not just because of their sex lives, but because they are powerless to act on decisions about their health.

> Therefore, orthodox behaviour change communication designed to influence individual sexual behaviour is not adequate for enabling sex workers to adopt safe sexual practices. Sex workers are handicapped because they are socially excluded by the combination of their class, gender and sexuality, and by the moral stigmatisation caused by their profession . . . Structural social rules exclude them materially and their stigmatisation adds to their material deprivation. Given these conditions sex workers as a group will have to be enabled to break through the structural barriers that keep them excluded from access to resources as well as participation in society before any individual sex worker can be really empowered to protect herself.
>
> (Jana et al., 1999)

A very important founding principle was that the issue of HIV among prostitutes was framed in terms of improving occupational safety and health (Jana et al., 2004). Accordingly, the prostitutes were called 'sex-workers' and their status shifted discursively from immoral criminals to being a part of the local economy. This enduring aspect of the programme has reduced the stigmatization of sex workers and increased their expectation of their own rights. It has also defined HIV prevention as a community issue and in the economic interests of all stakeholders.

Objectives

The overall objective of the programme is to reduce the incidence of STIs and HIV/AIDS among the sex workers. However, its broader health benefits are part of the success of the programme and the aims now include a broader conceptualization of well being. Jana et al. (2004) describe the key components of the programme as providing objectives that are transferable to other HIV prevention programmes:

1 Redefining the problem in a way that does not stigmatize individuals.
2 Helping the community assume responsibility by highlighting benefits for all.
3 Reducing environmental barriers to implementation.
4 Providing resources.

Theoretical model for intervention

The project developers describe the principles behind the development of this participatory programme as a model for 'creating an enabling environment' (Jana et al., 1999). These basic principles are described as:

1 No attempt to 'rescue' or 'rehabilitate' sex workers. Their capabilities as human beings and workers were recognized and respected as a commitment by organizers to *respect* sex work and persons engaged in sex work, to *rely* on them to run the programme, and to *recognize* their professional and human rights.
2 Sex workers were not treated as passive 'beneficiaries' but as *change agents*.
3 Sex workers were regarded as persons with a range of emotional and material needs and not merely in terms of their sexual behaviour.
4 Sex workers' own needs and interests were given prime importance in designing and carrying out any activity.
5 Emphasis on genuine representation and active participation of the sex workers at every level of the programme.

Implementation

The guiding principles have been translated into practice at three levels of community activity: working with the sex workers, working with the controllers of the sex trade, and working at advocacy and policy level as described by Jana et al. (1999):

1 *Working with the community of sex workers.*
   ♦ Trust was developed between the programme managers and the sex workers by involving them in all aspects of planning and implementation of programme components.
   ♦ Activities that directly addressed the needs articulated by sex workers such as literacy training, and services for sex workers' children were undertaken whether they matched the goals of the managers or not.
   ♦ Sex workers' contributions and role as workers were highlighted at local, national and international forums to make them visible as legitimate citizens, and to inculcate pride and worthiness.
   ♦ Steps were taken against all discriminatory practices, within the sex trade (police harassment, violence, oppression by madams, etc.) and outside it (exclusion of their children from education, social stigma, etc.).
   ♦ These activities increased capacity and self-esteem and empowered workers socially, economically and politically.
2 *Working with the controllers of the sex trade.*
   ♦ Acceptance of prostitution as a valid profession reassured other stakeholders in the sex trade that outsiders would not disrupt their business.
   ♦ Each red light area was studied to map the relation of power and conflicts of interest between groups of stakeholders in the sex industry. Using these understandings, strategies were evolved to develop support within the sex trade.
   ♦ Special activities were targeted at madams, pimps and regular clients, to orient them to the risk of transmission of HIV and to the larger programme objectives, encouraging them to work with the programme.
3 *Advocacy to influence policy.* Extensive and ongoing advocacy campaigns and individual lobbying were undertaken to persuade opinion leaders and policymakers of the legitimacy of the approach and entitlement of sex workers to equal rights. Local opinion makers, elected representatives, ministers, political party officials, human rights and other democratic fronts, women's groups, trade unions, bureaucrats, intellectuals, other NGOs, donor agencies, international HIV related networks and others were targeted. Consequently, the Sonagachi Project gained public recognition, wide acceptance and opportunities to carry out more radical changes. The committee was also able to use this credibility to question and challenge some fundamental structural constraints that exclude sex workers from policy consideration and social participation.
4 *The programme.* Empowerment through knowledge and tools for health are the centre of this programme. Peer educators provide sexual health education to sex workers and madams, and distribute condoms. Many STI/HIV clinics in and around the red light areas offer treatment to sex workers and their children. In wider development components, women may attend literacy classes taught by other sex workers, and enrol their

children in daycare, school and other programmes at special educational centres. To foster economic security, a community lending cooperative (Usha Multipurpose Cooperative Society) provides affordable loans and has over 5000 members. The Sonagachi Project also promotes the talents of sex workers through a cultural wing – The Komal Gandhar. In addition, an antitrafficking unit controlled by self-regulatory boards works across West Bengal to protect children and provide homes.

Participation is a key feature. In 1995, the sex worker community served by the project developed the DMSC network and created forums dealing with basic rights to health in the broader framework of livelihood security and self-determination. DMSC took over management of the project in 1999. The group advocates for the rights and interests of sex workers, and leads a movement to decriminalize prostitution (see The Communication Initiative, 2004).

Conclusions

Success has been shown in terms of AIDS prevalence and development. Jana et al. (2004) cite evidence showing that among sex workers condom use is higher, and HIV seroprevalence and infection rates among sex workers is lower in Calcutta than in other Indian cities. Shyamali Gupta, president of the All India Democratic Women's Association in West Bengal said about Songachi:

> The instances of oppression by pimps and policemen have come down drastically. The women are now aware of their rights and they want the next generation to have a better life. Their children can now use their mothers' names to get admitted in schools. Moreover, thanks to many vocational courses, the women are becoming more productive with their lives outside their profession.
>
> (Chattopadhyay, 2005)

Community capacity building using community resources

The four projects described in this section draw on participatory principles to draw upon and develop community capacity. In ways that are both similar and different across the contexts for the interventions, the project partners are interested in drawing on the expertise, knowledge and talents within communities of people, and developing new confidence and awareness of their capacity to improve their lives and health. Accordingly, although there are no specific illnesses or diseases targeted in these projects, the community members are seen as disadvantaged and lacking in the material and social resources that promote health. Such projects are often understood as addressing inequalities through the support and development of disadvantaged communities.

A community participatory project in Canada to promote child health

The Highfield Community Enrichment Project was one of eight sites for a broader, community-wide initiative in primary prevention and health promotion for young children living in a low income suburb of Toronto, Ontario (Nelson et al., 2005).

Evidence and theoretical basis for understanding the health issue

The overarching programme, Better Beginnings Better Futures, is a government ministry funded programme designed to test the efficacy of community-based primary prevention and health promotion policy. The evidence driving this government policy suggested that health and social problems will be prevented by strengthening the health of children, families and the community (Nelson et al., 2004), and that the best primary prevention programmes have a high level of community involvement (Pancer et al., 2003).

Objectives

The three major goals of this overarching programme were:

1 The prevention of problems in young children.
2 The promotion of competence and health of young children.
3 Strengthening vulnerable families and communities.

Theoretical model for intervention

The Highfield project is based on a participatory model in which participation is conceptualized in terms of two important concepts: partnership and empowerment (Nelson et al., 2004).

1 Partnership is seen in terms of three steps that should precede project goals.
    ♦ Forming the partnership by identifying key stakeholders and creating a forum for them to come together.
    ♦ Deciding the values of the partnership. Open consideration of the values such as collaboration and power sharing underlying the partnership is a critical step.
    ♦ Identifying and valuing the different strengths of the partners. All types of knowledge, including scientific, professional and local experience are pooled on an equal footing.
2 Empowerment is seen as the philosophy that guides value-based partnerships.
    ♦ Empowering processes provide real opportunities for participation.
    ♦ Empowered outcomes are increased control of resources for disadvantaged community members.

Implementation

The Highfield School neighbourhood is densely populated with a high percentage of single parents and families on low incomes. Nearly 60 percent of the population was born outside Canada. The Highfield Community Enrichment Project partnerships were first developed in making a proposal for funding to the government programme. A core group of seven service providers (education, social services and health) and one community resident submitted the project proposal. A needs survey of the community and a follow up meeting of residents led to three areas of project focus: in-school programmes, family support and community development. Once funded, a project manager and staff were hired. This project planning and start up phase took more than two years.

Following funding, the project was managed by an executive group whose membership has included at least four residents, one of whom chaired the team. There were also three subcommittees of the executive team who made most decisions at the programme level, and residents formed a significant proportion of these committees. Other community members acted as parent volunteers, in classroom programmes and in the family resource centre. Some volunteers found employment on the project. An important aspect of developing opportunities for participation has been in material support such as providing childcare for all meetings.

There were many activities undertaken within the three areas of project focus. Among the classroom focused programmes were a social skills programme implemented by teachers, and a health and nutrition programme in which healthy snacks and hot lunches were provided. An important component was the employment of educational assistants and parent volunteers as enrichment workers in the classroom to assist with academic, social and language skill building. Family support programmes were provided by a family resource centre with drop-in mornings, playgroups and a toy lending library. Home visitors for families with young children also connected young children with the school. Community focused programmes included celebrations, breakfasts, barbecues and ethnocultural events. Before and after school recreational programmes for neighbourhood children, and language and vocational skills for older children were provided (Pancer et al., 2003).

Conclusion

The project has undergone comprehensive evaluation as part of the original proposal (Nelson et al., 2004). Members of the research group conclude that the project is a successful example of a cost-effective approach to preventing child problems (as opposed to treating them once they arise). The evaluation results are particularly encouraging in regard to reducing the stress and improving childcare and social skills of parents.

A community participatory project in Australia to promote child health

Campbell et al. (2007) provide a critical account of a participatory community development strategy with indigenous people in Australia. A very remote town of 750 Aboriginal people (from 12 different descent groups) is characterized by very low levels of income, employment and education in comparison with non-Aboriginal Australia. Health is poor and this project was concerned with the health of children. This account is based on their paper.

Evidence and theoretical basis for understanding the health issue

The Department of Health and Community services (DHCS) in the Northern Territory of Australia introduced a growth assessment and action policy for rural Aboriginal children. Research had shown poorer health and poor growth or low weight for these children.

DCHS health professionals subsequently identified programme deficiencies including insufficient involvement of Aboriginal people, poor understanding by service providers of social and cultural issues, and lack of guidelines for promoting community growth promotion action. Meanwhile, a group of Aboriginal women from a remote community had discussed their concerns about child growth and agreed to collaborate with DHCS on a child growth community oriented project.

Objectives

The objectives for the project were:

1 Improve child growth by increasing community action.
2 Inform the broader growth action programme by documenting Aboriginal perceptions of child growth and the process of community action.

Theoretical model for intervention

The project was based on a community development model which includes understandings of participation and empowerment.

Participation in community development for health promotion involves supporting groups to identify their health issues, and then plan and implement strategies for change. Ownership and definition of the problems and the solutions is the basis of a participatory community development approach. Because the community members had identified poor child growth as a concern, this project appeared to be beginning with these first principles of a participatory process. These participatory processes are seen as empowering. As well as the opportunity to change outcomes, people gain increased self-reliance and decision making abilities as a result of their activities. Empowerment is understood to contribute to improved individual and collective health status in its own right as people gain greater control over their lives.

This community development model is considered a useful strategy in addressing Aboriginal health issues. 'It is strongly supported by Aboriginal leaders and Aboriginal controlled health services and is consistent with Aboriginal demands for greater control over their affairs' (Campbell et al., 2007, p. 152).

A participatory action research framework was used as the basis for study because of the emphasis on locally defined priorities and perspectives and the sharing of power between all participants, which fits with the development approach. This framework involved an ongoing spiral of planning, action and reflection by analysing data and feeding back key findings to participants throughout the project.

Implementation

The project was funded by the DHCS and a research centre for Aboriginal health. The health professionals working in the local DHCS clinic were an important part of the programme. A (non-Aboriginal) project leader consulted with community members for 18 months and then designed the Child Growth Project with the project officer (non-Aboriginal development worker). An Aboriginal project adviser and two co-workers were recruited locally and worked closely with the project officer.

Data were collected at different stages throughout the project using semi-structured interviews in respondents' first language, group discussions, photovoice, participant observation and recording of children's weights from their medical charts at health clinic visits. The findings were fed back through posters, reports, community meetings, the local radio station and a video.

This comprehensive feedback process resulted in a shift in the identified problem. Local people were more concerned about poor childcare, nutrition and development (rather than illness as being a cause of small size). A committee of Aboriginal community members developed a strategy they named a Family Centre and this aspect of the project has continued to be implemented with support from the project team and further government funding. The Family Centre is a multifaceted strategy designed to promote childcare and development through a playgroup, early childhood education (including Aboriginal law and culture), preparing children for mainstream schooling, educating parents about care for children, growth monitoring and promotion activities run by clinic staff, and after school activities for teenagers.

Conclusion

The development of this approach was hampered by health care professionals who did not agree with the shift from a focus on physical growth (which they saw as caused by illness only) to a focus on child development and family support. Non-Aboriginal clinic staff did not support the Family Centre strategy, although many Aboriginal parents did not attend the clinic and little data was collected about child growth in that domain. Health professionals were unwilling to relinquish control and their own definition of the health problem. Although this resistance hampered the development of the project, local community members were able to take control of the issue and develop their own strategy. Campbell et al. (2007) provide a detailed evaluation of this aspect of the process to which we will return in Chapter 8.

A community arts project to promote fish harvester safety in Canada

Another Canadian project used community participation in a different way. Commercial fishing, on which many Newfoundland communities depend, is a very dangerous occupation. Health promoters engaged with the local fishing communities' cultural traditions to raise awareness of safety issues and develop a safety culture (Murray and Tilley, 2006).

Evidence and theoretical basis for understanding the health issue

Murray and Tilley (2006) provide evidence to explain the dangers of fishing to life and limb. Current occupational health and safety research includes the importance of a safety culture (a shift from individual perceptions to a collective approach). There is evidence that lack of a safety culture contributes to high rates of accidents in the fishing industry.

Objectives

The broad aim of a planned intervention was to explore methods to promote a safety culture not to provide more knowledge about safety issues (fish harvesters undertake formal safety training), but to raise community awareness of their importance (Murray and Tilley, 2005).

Theoretical model for intervention

In organizational theory there is a shift from 'top–down' management driven efforts, toward a 'bottom–up approach' to developing a safety culture, which considers the power relations between workers and management. These understandings naturally extend to the broader context of workers' lives and to a community approach to safety which has been successfully used in Scandinavia and elsewhere (Murray and Tilley, 2005). This approach uses the strengths of all people involved to make changes in awareness, behaviour and environment.

An important community strength is in culture and arts. This is the basis of a community arts approach to health promotion which draws on the heritage and resources of a community. Arts may engage many community members in ways that can promote shared understandings and transformation of issues of concern.

Principles of community action were drawn on to encourage community control and ownership of the programme. The focus on fishery safety and the use of arts-based activities was chosen by the project leaders. The actual details of the programme were developed in collaboration with community residents.

Implementation

The project was conducted in three fishing communities in Newfoundland. The project leaders (community development workers and health promotion researchers) saw themselves as facilitators and contributed knowledge of safety issues, while the community participants developed the programme content based on local interest, culture, skills and talent. Thus, the programme was developed differently in each community.

Community A had a population of 4145. An advisory committee of fishermen, fish plant workers, local teachers and artists provided ongoing advice. A local person was employed to coordinate activities and issue press releases. There were various activities including writing, drama, graphic arts and song writing. These were showcased in Fishery Safety Week through an ecumenical church service, safety demonstrations, art displays and a community concert. The concert included readings of poems and short stories about safety at sea by students, songs presented by two local groups and the school choir and orchestra, and a play about safety in the fishery especially written and performed by members of the local community. Money raised at these events was donated to a memorial fund.

Community B, with a total population of about 1500, centred the programme around a local theatre group with local actors. The group's administrator acted as coordinator for the project, and the artistic director arranged arts activities. An advisory committee additionally included local fish harvesters, school teachers and a member of the harbour authority. Teachers initiated activities in the school. A series of cultural activities was planned around Fishing Safety Week. The theatre group performed a play dealing with the drowning of fishermen, which was accompanied by traditional music and song. Children's drawings about safety at sea were displayed on the walls. These activities were reported in the local newspaper.

Community C had a population of about 960. An advisory committee comprised the mayor, local fish harvesters and a fish processor. A coordinator was appointed and although there is no school, the town has an active youth committee, which expressed interest in the activities. A video was developed, in which the mayor and six fish harvesters described their views and the impact of a disaster on a family and the community. A breakfast meeting was held to show and discuss the video and safety issues in general. A dinner and dance was held in the community centre at which the video was also shown along with other presentations about community responsibility for safety. A special church service was held at which four local church ministers blessed the fishing fleet along with readings and songs.

Conclusion

All of these events were beset by various issues and problems, as might be expected (see Murray and Tilley, 2005). However, members of all communities expressed enthusiasm for the events, their raised awareness of safety issues and their enjoyment of the activities. The project showed that it is possible to engage large numbers of people from various parts of a community in activities concerned with safety.

Participation and empowerment to reduce health inequalities in Brazil

Guareschi and Jovchelovitch (2004) have described the ongoing development of participatory practices in Porto Alegre, a large city in Brazil. Porto Alegre has implemented a democratic system of participatory budgeting based on citizen forums and thematic meetings that is related to improvements in sanitation, housing, health and education over the last 12 years. Nevertheless, there are wide inequalities in the city. In the context of a participatory political setting, Guareschi and Jovchelovitch describe the theoretical basis for developing participatory projects aimed at empowerment to reduce inequalities and this account is taken from their paper.

Evidence and theoretical basis for understanding the health issue

These authors note that it is now generally understood that the health of the poor can only be understood within the broader context of general conditions of living. In their own experience, working in the *vilas* (extremely deprived squatter communities) of Brazil, participatory projects have repeatedly shown that for the poor, health is part of a set of practices involving basic conditions such as sanitation, electricity, waste collection and disposal, housing, education, transport, security and leisure. Thus, health is not an abstract notion but knowledge about how health and illness is lived in daily life. Poor people face concrete lack of resources and develop strategies for living through and improving their situation. Participation for empowerment is one of these strategies.

Objectives

The objectives of the programme are to reduce inequalities by incorporating the demands of the poor into health policies. Guareschi and Jovelovitch

Questions

1 On what levels did the intervention conceptualize and approach the issues?
2 Was the intervention theoretically coherent across the stages of development?
3 How was the theoretical framework applied to the aspects of the intervention?
4 What are the different ways in which community and participation are defined or operationalized? What are the similarities and differences between the different approaches?
5 Who got to participate in any particular project? Which people may have been advantaged and who may have been missed or excluded?
6 What are the values behind the choices made by the practitioners?
7 What ethical issues can you highlight in each of these interventions?

Many of the issues raised by reflecting on the planning, implementation and outcomes of an intervention suggest questions that will be answered through formal evaluation research. The ongoing evaluation of health promotion activities is one of the main ways that we have for understanding the effects of our practices. Formal evaluation research is outlined and discussed in the next chapter.

CHAPTER
8

Evaluation of health promotion programmes

Introduction

Evaluation of health promotion activities is essential to assess their success and to monitor the ethical implications of all aspects of interventions. During health promotion activities many different questions arise about the effects of the work. Has our health promotion intervention made any difference to people's health? Who has benefited from the intervention? How do the participants understand the activities? Have we done any harm? These kinds of intuitively obvious questions immediately demonstrate not just the need for evaluation, but also the range of evaluative questions that may be asked. As the importance of formal evaluation of any intervention programme has gained increasing recognition (not least because funding bodies want to know that their money has been used for good purpose and are increasingly prepared to fund evaluation research) the science of evaluation has developed as an area of theorizing and methodology in its own right. And, like any area of serious activity, there are debates and controversies regarding theory and methodology appropriate to evaluation activities (e.g., Wimbush and Watson, 2000; Burton et al., 2006; Tucker et al., 2006).

In this chapter I do not wish to engage in these debates, but rather to point to some useful ways that have been developed to broadly structure the range of evaluation activities in health promotion, and to consider some of the substantive and methodological issues that are raised by the shift toward complex, community and participatory health promotion programmes. In doing so, I will consider three different aspects of evaluation that have been identified by various researchers as: formative evaluation (front end planning); process evaluation (functioning of the programme activities); and outcome evaluation (the planned end results). Of course, there are overlaps between evaluation issues across these three aspects, and the move from planning to process to outcomes is not necessarily straightforward at all. Here, I will discuss formative, then outcome and, finally, process issues. I have chosen this order because a shift towards community-based and participatory theories and models, has resulted in recent shifts in emphasis from the importance of long-term outcomes to a much greater interest in the effects of everyday processes as a valued aspect of health promotion.

Formative evaluation

Ideally, an evaluation plan is an integral part of the intervention planning. This means that every objective, every specific aim, each theoretical construct that is part of the intervention design is already a clearly specified target for evaluation. Evaluation takes into account every step of the planning from decisions about the health issues and consideration of the theoretical targets for change, through to the models and methods used, and how all these steps are related to the desired outcomes. Adams et al. (2007) describe the importance of the evaluation of these planning stages which they call 'formative evaluation' or 'front end'. They describe the evaluation of the intervention planning itself as a process to ensure that there are strong links between the objectives, strategies and activities. This aspect of evaluation is designed to ensure that effective strategies will be used to meet the specified programme objectives.

Planning as an integral part of evaluation

The design and development of intervention programmes is integral to their evaluation. A number of models have been developed to support systematic consideration of this planning. Wimbush and Watson (2000) list examples of such models from several countries and note that these models share similar understandings of the key stages and the different evaluation focus of each stage. 'Intervention mapping' is another tool which has been proposed by Kok et al. (2004) to systematically assist the planning for prevention interventions. Such planning uses theory and evidence to specify the needs, health issues, population, programme objectives and methods for implementing the plan. Each of these specifications becomes a target for evaluation at each step of the programme. The mapping as proposed by these authors emphasizes the importance of theory in developing objectives for evaluation and provides for the careful consideration of the goals of the intervention before, during and after implementation. Such a well specified plan is very well suited to non-participatory designs, in which the programme leaders are the experts who choose the issues, theory and intervention methods. As a general approach that emphasizes specifically articulated and discussed goals, it is an excellent model for any evaluation plan. However, in participatory and complex community led health promotion programmes, there are some additional issues and hurdles to consider.

Issues in community and participatory approaches

In participatory research designs, participation may be one important goal, but outcome objectives, such as particular health needs to be met, are not necessarily well developed at the beginning of the programme. Indeed, as part of any participatory process, goals often shift, the goals of different partners may be at odds or they may change as part of the partnership development. Community designs are often complex with longer time frames, and the evaluation design must fit with the local context which necessarily varies from programme to programme. Kemp et al. (2007) point to some of these issues in the context of programmes whose aims are to assist the development of economically disadvantaged communities and improve health. Given the current evidence that the strength of community is a determinant of health, many such development programmes have been recently implemented. Kemp et al. draw on two examples of work in disadvantaged communities in Australia to consider four questions (p. 2):

◆ Are we doing what we say we are doing?
◆ Are we measuring what we say we are doing?
◆ Are we measuring what we say we are measuring?
◆ Are we introducing evidence-based practice for which there is no evidence?

They conclude by suggesting that programme developers and evaluators must consider the roles of local context and develop more critical considerations of the links between intervention, evaluation and community outcomes within particular community contexts.

Formative evaluation in community practice

Adams et al. (2007) conducted an evaluation of a community programme in New Zealand that was designed to address the social determinants of health inequalities. This intervention was based in theories of social capital and social cohesion as pathways to reduction in health inequalities. Because this evaluation was funded by two government agencies which brought in external evaluators, the community representatives were initially resistant to the value of the evaluation project. Accordingly, an evaluation plan was negotiated and community representatives were included in a group formed to guide and critique the evaluation activities. The formative evaluator conducted a needs assessment, developed a community profile, and assessed the links between the programme objectives, strategies and activities. The evaluators found that there was a tension between the immediate demands for evidence of success and the long-term goals of the project. There was an early rush to develop many small participatory projects, which were beyond the organizers' capacity to monitor and strategic planning was slow to develop. This aspect of the evaluation revealed both programme strengths and barriers to strategic planning and implementation. For example, the slow development of planning skills, and problems of cohesion among groups of participants, was a barrier. These findings were seen as contributing to the development of the project as part of an action research cycle of planning, implementing and reviewing.

Community programme developers are developing specific tools to assist in the formative evaluation process. In the US, Ndirangu et al. (2007) described the use of a 'comprehensive participatory planning and evaluation' (CPPE) model to identify community needs in a participatory project. This planning model is based on the principles of context driven development, and the role of the community in setting priorities, planning and implementing strategies for health promotion. Ndirangu et al. applied this model to conduct a needs assessment in a rural community with previously identified health issues, such as high rates of disease. According to their assessment of its use, the model allowed community and university partners to learn from each other and contribute equally as opposed to a 'top–down' decision making process. Community members helped to define the research agenda and identified interventions that they felt would assist in their local setting. The authors also identified three limitations to this planning process: the sacrifice of time to contribute placed a high demand on community members and excluded many; the need for a certain level of literacy to participate excluded many; and some priorities were raised by community members that were not within the mandate of the university partners to address. In other words, these issues severely limited participation and raised questions regarding the final decision making power of the different partners in such a project. One of the important benefits of conducting such evaluations is that these issues are highlighted for consideration, rather than being hidden behind broad claims of community participation.

One of the important issues raised in the formative evaluation of community-based programmes is the need for flexibility related to local context, and the need for time for the careful development of relationships and negotiated objectives. These issues are theoretically addressed within an action research paradigm in which evaluation is not imposed upon the participants, but is a central aspect of the conceptualization of programme development. The principles of action research as originally set out by Lewin (1997, p. 146) as 'a circle of planning, action, and fact-finding about the result of the action' have been increasingly drawn upon and developed for application in community based participatory health related programmes (see Minkler and Wallerstein, 2003).

Formative evaluation involves consideration of the planning of any intervention programme including the development of programme goals and the ways that these goals are linked with activities and outcomes. It has probably gained more importance as an aspect of evaluation in the context of very complex, context related, long-term projects. At the same time, the complexity and participatory nature of these projects raises a number of issues regarding how planning activities themselves are carried out and who gets to make decisions about goals and activities. Community researchers are rapidly developing a range of tools and approaches to deal with these issues and the principles of action research are providing an important basis for many of these developments. In general, evaluation of the formative activities of any health related intervention requires initial, ongoing, reflexive attention to the theoretical and ethical issues that have been raised across each chapter of this book.

Outcome evaluation

Outcomes have been focused on by programme designers and funders as the point and purpose of any intervention. The important evaluation question has traditionally been seen as unequivocally related to behaviour changes and positive health changes that result from an intervention: 'following our programme, has the target population changed their diet to include more healthy foods, or has there been a decrease in heart disease?' These kinds of questions have also proved to be the most difficult to answer. Consequently many theoretical and methodological approaches have been proposed to address the various issues raised regarding outcome evaluation. One of the first aspects to consider is what outcomes are expected in terms of a programme's objectives. This question has produced some attempts to structure our thinking about what we should expect.

Structuring observation of outcomes

Any programme is expected to produce different sorts of outcomes across time in what has been called a 'proximal–distal chain of effects' (Wimbush and Watson, 2000). This notion suggests a series of effects across time, with one outcome expected to impact on another. Many evaluation researchers use the terms proximal (immediate changes) and distal (down the track changes that are expected to follow) to differentiate these types of outcomes. Nutbeam (1998) describes these outcomes across time in terms of three different levels:

♦ Health promotion outcomes (proximal). These are seen as the immediate changes that are expected to affect determinants of health. For example, attitudes and beliefs that are theorized to affect behaviour, motivation to take up healthy lifestyles, empowerment and capacity of community members to make changes, or the development of social capital.
♦ Intermediate health outcomes (distal). These are outcomes theorized to

follow from the proximal changes. They could include improved personal behaviours such as increased exercise or reduced tobacco use; healthier environments, which allow for physical activity or improve material conditions; access to appropriate health services; or social cohesion.

♦ Health and social outcomes (most distal). These might include improved quality of life, equity, changes in disease experience, illness incidence, or physical and mental health in the population.

The brief examples included here are chosen to make the point that the outcomes expected at each stage of a chain of effects may vary widely, and the particular outcome expected will depend upon the theory of health and health promotion that is being drawn upon. Below, I will develop some examples of the kinds of proximal and distal outcomes that may be considered.

Proximal outcomes

Proximal outcomes are the changes that are expected as a direct result of any intervention or programme. Models based on social cognitive theories, such as the theory of planned behaviour, provide very clearly specified targets for change. These include changes in the cognitive determinants of behaviour such as attitudes, beliefs or knowledge, and these are usually measured in the individuals (or samples of the population) who are expected to change. To assess this change, specific proximal outcomes of an intervention based on these kinds of theories may be measured in the population before and after any intervention. The methods used to evaluate these outcomes are usually quantitative and questionnaire-based, and the ideal has been experimental including random assignment to intervention or control groups.

An example of a carefully developed and evaluated health promotion intervention is provided by SHARE. This is a sexual education programme for Scottish adolescents, based on the theory of planned behaviour and sociological theorizing to explain young people's sexual behaviours and protective practices. The programme was applied to sex education in schools and evaluated across several stages of its operation (see Abraham et al., 1998; Wight et al., 1998; Wight and Abraham, 2000). The impact of the programme on targeted cognitions was tested using a randomized controlled trial which compared the SHARE results with those of conventional sex education programmes across a number of schools. Those receiving SHARE were more likely to believe that there were alternatives to sexual intercourse in romantic relationships; more likely to intend to resist unwanted sexual relationships and discuss condoms with partners; and had more positive attitudes to condom use. However, these differences were small, and there were no differences in important intentions such as to always use a condom (Abraham et al., 2004).

More complex socially based theories of health have moved away from a focus on individual cognitions as the basis of health behaviour. Focus on theories of the social basis of health has introduced notions such as empowerment, capacity and social capital as the primary objectives of community-based interventions. Nutbeam (1998) describes the purpose of health promotion activity as strengthening the skills and capabilities of individuals so that they can control the determinants of health. Thus, capacity and empowerment are the valued outcomes. Socially based approaches have also included changes in evaluation approaches. In terms of methods, evaluators have included more in depth qualitative research to evaluate the initial outcomes.

For example, the aims of a complex community development programme in New Zealand (Adams et al., 2007) included the development of neighbourhood cohesion as a pathway to improved health outcomes. Consequently, an initial evaluation of outcomes focused on measures of social cohesion. The chief instrument for this assessment was a before and after survey of neighbourhood cohesion. This survey was undertaken at the behest of the funders, however, the evaluators were cautious about the value of developing survey items before community strategic planning was completed and about the value of attributing change over time with this sort of methodology. In regard to the first issue, they were concerned to review specific outcomes once the project aims had been developed, and to use key informant interview data to complement the survey results. Once the survey and interviews were aligned, they found that interview data complemented initial survey results by providing explanations of outcomes in particular areas where tensions and issues were revealed, and increased the value of the survey data in the eyes of the stakeholders. The most important aspect of the evaluation findings in the first three years of the project was to inform its ongoing development and the reflective practices of the team.

Pérez et al. (2007) evaluated a community participatory project in Cuba whose overarching objective was to prevent dengue fever. These evaluators used a sociological analysis with qualitative data to assess the effectiveness of the programme. They concluded that the success of this project lay in a shift on the part of the project team, from viewing participation as just one component in the prevention strategy to recognizing its fundamental importance as a learning and empowering process for the participants. They suggest that to be successful, community-based prevention must be a social learning process with real transfer of power and responsibilities to local people. Similarly, a community development project in India was evaluated in terms of its success in contributing to gender development and the empowerment, capability and participation of women (Tesoriero, 2006). Women's self-help groups were found to make a ('modest but significant') contribution towards transformations of oppressive structures. Wallerstein (2006) has reviewed the evidence from evaluations of such empowerment strategies to provide a set of clear suggestions for future actions by health promoters.

Distal outcomes

The health and social well being outcomes that are expected to eventuate from health promotion are the most difficult to evaluate. Adams et al. (2007) were concerned about their ability to attribute any observed population changes in proximal outcomes to a broad-based intervention. Making final attributions regarding health outcomes, often several years down the track, has proved to be an even more difficult task. Tucker et al. (2006) note that although there are increasing demands for health promotion activities to show effects on health outcomes, demonstrating attributable effect is extremely difficult in practice. Wallerstein (2006) also notes that linking community and psychological empowerment to health has been difficult. Many interventions do not deliver the hoped for changes and it is easier to find examples of failure in individual studies and systematic reviews of evaluation research rather than success.

For example, the SHARE project described above has been the object of more distal outcome evaluations after two years. Wight et al. (2002) described a randomly controlled trial of areas in Scotland in which school pupils had or had not received the SHARE programme. The study compared baseline and follow up questionnaire responses from 8430 pupils to assess the study's aim of reducing unsafe sexual intercourse by measuring exposure to sexually transmitted disease, use of condoms and unwanted pregnancies. The results showed that although the SHARE pupils had better knowledge and attitudes to sexual behaviour, there were no differences between the groups in sexual activity, sexual risk taking or unwanted pregnancies.

Tucker et al. (2006) suggest that the reasons for such difficulties may include the design of interventions, time lag effects, potential intervening and confounding factors, and the high cost of good evaluation research for large scale interventions. The movement towards complex community-based and participatory programmes, raises even more issues. Merzel and D'Afflitti (2003) reviewed the outcomes across two decades of a variety of community health promotion programmes in the US. They conclude that 'achieving behavioural and health change across an entire community is a challenging goal that many programmes have failed to attain'. They suggest several factors that contribute to the modest impact of such interventions (the most successful being HIV prevention programmes). These include both methodological limitations in the evaluation research, and limited scope of the interventions themselves. Many programmes still focus on individual change and use single approaches such as mass education. Many of the more difficult aims such as developing community capacity and larger social economic and political forces, are not addressed. We will turn now to consider suggestions for grappling with these issues including the evaluation methods, aims and actual processes of health promotion programmes.

Issues in outcome evaluation

When considering the failure of health promotion interventions in many areas of behavioural, disease state, or social change, three central questions are often discussed. Are we using appropriate methods to evaluate health related outcomes? Are we choosing appropriate outcomes as our objectives? What actually happened during the intervention that impacted on the outcomes? I will consider these questions in turn below.

Are the methods appropriate?

Tucker et al. (2006) have reviewed recent debates in the literature regarding the negative findings from randomized controlled trials, pointing to suggestions that such findings have arisen from flawed evaluation methods which are mistimed, misplaced or use inappropriate measures of behaviour or outcome. Nutbeam (1998) has considered additional issues raised by disappointing results from carefully evaluated large scale community level interventions in which there are no differences between intervention groups and other populations. It is not that there have been no gains, rather that all groups have improved their behaviours or health outcomes. Such observed changes seem to arise from the long-term development of social movements rather than from focused interventions. He has noted that the most powerful and effective forms of health promotion, in other words, those that are capable of addressing complex social and economic determinants of health, are less easily predicted, controlled and measured with traditional methods. Nutbeam recommends the inclusion of qualitative methods to examine some of these more complex social changes. In developing an evaluation of a sexual health programme for young people in Scotland (which includes the ongoing SHARE education programme), Tucker et al. (2006) also propose the advantages of methodological pluralism: a combination of qualitative and quantitative measures. While recognizing some inherent limitiations in this approach (and the limitations of political and social forces beyond the programme) they describe its advantages. Like Adams et al. (2007) they consider the usefulness of complementary methods, which are able to consider and explain different aspects of the process and outcome aspects of a programme as they interact together. Changing methodological approaches in this way enables moves toward including the importance of process, not simply as accounting for practical matters that may hamper a desired outcome, but as a critical aspect of the ongoing impact of any programme on its participants. Methods of evaluation must be closely related to the impact of an intervention in all of its aspects. Both qualitative and quantitive approaches to measurement are able to provide pieces of the puzzle and allow ongoing reflection on the direction of programme strategies. Considering intervention processes and outcomes as closely interrelated in this way raises our next issue: who decides which particular outcomes are valued?

Are we choosing appropriate outcomes?

Nutbeam (1998) has said that 'At its core evaluation concerns assessment of the extent to which an action achieves a *valued* outcome' (p. 28). There are many different interpretations of outcomes, and reflexive practice must consider the outcomes that are valued in any particular community health promotion programme. As the focus of health promotion moves towards employing socially based theories of health, community-based interventions focus on broader objectives such as empowerment and social cohesion. These are not the traditional disease related outcomes of a medically oriented public health within which conventional evaluation approaches and expectations have been developed. And yet, current evaluation practices tend to direct programme developers towards considering such broad theoretical notions as objects which may be operationalized for measurement and reported upon in terms of behavioural change.

Another issue arises here because of the shift towards valuing participation. If participatory processes are used to choose valued outcomes, it may turn out that some people don't value changing their behaviour in ways expected by intervention designers. Experimental or economic evaluations with outcomes valued by particular stakeholders are not appropriate or effective in social contexts in which the outcomes themselves are socially developed. For example, Tucker et al. (2006) note that in studies of adolescent pregnancy prevention in which experimental designs have shown little effect, other measures of client satisfaction or good practice yield more positive results. It is very likely that these are the very outcomes that the young mothers themselves are interested in.

Buchanan (2006) addresses this as an ethical issue and suggests that a values-based approach is appropriate when considering which outcomes are important. Reflection upon the aims of health promotion would lead to researchers considering the extent to which the objectives fit with the health promotion values. Buchanan proposes a humanist model as providing an alternative set of outcomes. Humanism values personal integrity and meaning as a goal in people's lives. From this perspective, physical health may not be a primary goal. To support this suggestion, Buchanan uses examples of research which show that physical health does not bring happiness, while finding a sense of purpose in life does lead to better physical health. Thus, humanistic values provide an alternative way to consider the aims of health promotion. The importance of Buchanan's paper is its emphasis on the awareness of the underlying values of any health promoting activity, and how these values are reflected in the choices made about important outcomes.

What happened during the intervention?

In assessing why these projects do not deliver hoped for outcomes the process of the intervention must be taken into account. Campbell (2003) has described a community-based project whose main objective was to prevent HIV/AIDS by encouraging safer sex practices including the use of condoms and STI clinics. An outcome evaluation after three years of this project was conducted by epidemiologists and biomedical researchers in the form of quantitative surveys to measure biomedical, behavioural and social factors among a random sample of 2000 people each year. The results of initial data analysis showed that the project had no impact on levels of STIs. If the project had been successful in increasing condom use and STI services, then reductions in STIs were expected. In fact, in one study group there was an increase in infections. In the results of Campbell's qualitative evaluation of the project's process, she provides explanations for these failures and suggestions for future planners. Her suggestions, which will be considered in more detail in the next section, show that the processes of an intervention are an integral aspect of the outcomes.

Similarly, Visser et al. (2004) describe the evaluation of an HIV/AIDS prevention programme in South African schools. Following two years of a socially based HIV/AIDS and life skills education programme, an outcome evaluation survey showed that learners gained knowledge about HIV/AIDS and protective behaviour, but there were no changes in their attitudes to condom use, feelings of personal control or psychological well being. There was also no evidence of any behaviour changes, and some learners reported more sexual experience with no change in protective behaviour. Visser et al. also examined the processes involved in the programme implementation and uptake to show their involvement in this lack of success.

Despite the difficulties, there is no suggestion that health promoters and communities should not value outcomes such as greater condom use, fewer STIs or fewer AIDS infections (although this should not be taken for granted). However, sometimes, the problems with achieving these outcomes are better understood by careful consideration of the process, and valuing aspects of that process as important outcomes in their own right.

Process evaluation

Process evaluation focuses on the internal operations of a programme to assess its strengths and weaknesses (Patton, 1997). Process evaluation may be seen as gathering detailed information that will assist in linking specific intervention activities with the outcomes. Traditional evaluation research in health promotion has evaluated the processes of an intervention with questions such as, 'Did the intervention activities actually reach the target group?' 'Did the participants understand the materials?' or 'Was the programme delivered as planned?' For educational or mass media programmes that are based on individual change by education and persuasion, these are important questions. If the teachers do not deliver the classroom programme or the leaflets are not written in the common language, then it is these mechanical aspects of the intervention process that will prevent success.

Process evaluation in researcher led interventions

For an example of carefully conducted process evaluation we can return to the SHARE project which is described above. This theory-based, teacher delivered sex education programme was subjected to comprehensive evaluation of the processes involved at several steps throughout the development of the programme (Wight and Abraham, 2000). At the pilot stage, the teacher training was evaluated using participant observation, participants' questionnaires, and semistructured interviews. The resources for the classroom lessons were evaluated using teacher questionnaires, interviews with teachers and pupils, group discussions with pupils and observations of lessons. Comments were also sought from sex education experts and researchers. This research resulted in developing awareness for the designers regarding the practical and social constraints of a theory-based programme, and substantial changes to the materials. Most of the issues that arose were conflicts between the individual cognition basis of the theories, and the social and cultural situation of the classroom at many levels. For example, there were conflicts between the social-psychological knowledge on which the activities were based, and the accepted principles of current sex education practice among teachers. The lessons did not always fit with classroom culture, the experiences and social life of the students, or the needs and skills of the teachers. In recommending that such educational programmes must acknowledge and adapt to the sociocultural context of their application, Wight and Abraham (2000) suggest that 'this is likely to mean compromising some of the principles underlying the development of the intervention' (p. 35). This statement highlights the differences between social cognitive-theory-based approaches and socially oriented approaches. In the more individually based approach the sociocultural factors highlighted in the process evaluation were understood to have possible effects on the poor outcomes, and were controlled for in the analysis. They are extraneous variables. In community and participatory approaches, this sociocultural context is understood as essential to the process and outcomes of health promotion.

Process evaluation in community and participatory practice

Nutbeam (1998) has suggested the importance of the processes of an intervention in their own right, by drawing upon the principles of the Ottawa Charter in which health promotion is defined as '. . . the process of enabling people to exert control over the determinants of health and thereby improve their health' (p. 28). He includes this understanding of process as a valued aspect of health promotion activities. Evaluation of the processes of community approaches, based on these sorts of values, must go beyond the problems of delivery to include the complex contextual and multilevel social factors that are understood to impact on health and are also part of a health promoting programme. Visser et al. (2004) note that there is a lack of research about these complex social community processes in preventive interventions. Although, evaluators are beginning to take account of the social context, there are few conceptual frameworks that would enable planners to systematically address these processes.

A systems approach to process evaluation

Visser et al. (2004) evaluated a classroom-based sexual education programme in South Africa. They used interviews and focus group discussions, which were conducted with teachers, principals and learners across all the schools involved in the programme. Their process evaluation uncovered issues that were remarkably similar to those noted by the SHARE evaluators (Wight and Abraham, 2000). Problems in the delivery and uptake of the classroom lessons were located in the social context of the school situation. Visser et al. developed their analysis of the effects of these processes to show how they are an integral part of the disappointing outcomes of the intervention. To do this they applied systems theory to conceptualize the relationships between the processes and valued outcomes (which were for more protective sexual behaviour among young people).

A systems theory approach was used to develop a theoretical framework of four levels of social processes and a detailed analysis of the feedback and control processes between each. First order processes were defined as the interaction between learners resulting in safe sexual behaviour. Second order processes were defined as those which affect the first order. For example, education, which increases knowledge, or lack of effective education. Third order processes are exemplified by those that affect the organization in the school, including the principal and timetabling. Fourth order processes include broader social influences, such as the local community attitudes or educational institutional policy. Using this model, the analysis of the process evaluation data highlighted four important issues. The content of the programme was focused on knowledge, which is not well related to behaviour. The teachers were not well equipped to facilitate the extensive changes expected of the programme. There was no real participation by the local community, teachers and learners in the development of the programme, which was 'top–down' in a hierarchical fashion. The climate in the educational system and school community could not support the implementation. Visser et al. (2004) conclude that the capacity of the community to change and the various obstructive processes at each level of the system were not explored before the implementation of the programme. An analysis from a systems perspective highlights the basic importance and interconnection of social processes. Other theoretical perspectives include these social processes as valued aspects of the programme. Visser et al. highlighted the lack of participation across the social system. Evaluation from a participatory perspective foregrounds participation as an objective in its own right.

Participation as the focus for process evaluation

Nutbeam (1998) describes health promotion as a process that is directed towards enabling people to take action. Its purposes are strengthening the skills and capabilities of individuals. From this perspective, participatory processes are conceptualized as those that result in people being given power and control over their own outcomes. If power and control is the valued outcome, then participation is the key process. However, Estable et al. (2006) describe suggestions by evaluators that participatory research projects do not always achieve the participation that they intend.

Developing the evaluation of participation

Butterfoss (2006) has provided a review to describe how process evaluation has been used to determine success in achieving community participation. This review draws largely on the community-based participatory research (CBPR) literature, in which the action research cycle and participatory evaluation are fundamental methodologies. Butterfoss describes the methods that have been used to evaluate community participation in CBPR projects: participant surveys (standardized instruments have been developed to measure participation); event or activity logs (documenting the partnerships' accomplishments and actions); key informant interviews (with members, leaders and community stakeholders); focus groups (usually with members of the population served by the programme); and observations of meetings. The measures of participation used across these activities include a wide range of indicators such as the diversity of participants; the retention of members; the role of members in the activities; the number and type of events attended; the amount of time spent on coalition activities; benefits and challenges of participation; satisfaction with the work; and balance of power and leadership.

A community project in Istanbul, Turkey, used these sorts of indicators to evaluate participation. The Healthy Beginnings project (Turan et al., 2003) was developed with the aim of improving perinatal health for women in a densely populated district of Istanbul. Project activities were based in a community centre and the programme was initiated by a university team of researchers in child health – as an alternative to previously hospital-based antenatal education. The intervention was based on a ten-step community participation process, which aimed to involve community members in developing and delivering the educational objectives. Local women who had a personal interest in healthy child bearing joined the community team. Team members participated in regular meetings, site visits, small working groups and social events. To evaluate the success of the project in achieving community participation, five key indicators were selected from the literature: participation of the community group in decision making; gains in knowledge and skills of the community group; continuity of the community group; continuation of the health programme by the community group; and initiation of new support and advocacy activities by the target group. The results showed that community members participated in all decisions about group activities. Initially guided by project staff, the community members' decision making strengthened over time and community members became completely responsible for all course activities. They learned how to identify community problems and to design, implement and evaluate interventions to address those problems. After four years the meetings and activities of the group were continuing and the antenatal education course developed by the group continued to be successfully offered at the community centre. Course participants in turn have developed support networks and advocacy groups.

Increasingly formalized approaches to evaluation of participation clearly belong in the context of specific types of community partnerships. Other contexts may demand different sets of criteria and there are many different traditions in participatory evaluation. Springett (2003) notes that participatory evaluation may be seen as 'more a way of working based on a set of principles than an actual methodology' (p. 265). She notes the many approaches and labels used for participatory evaluation, while firmly placing its epistemology in the interpretivist tradition and the methodological roots in participatory action research. From this theoretical perspective, knowledge is created in practice between partners and on this basis, Springett describes the steps in an evaluation process which is participatory itself (p. 274):

1 All participants decide to use a participatory approach.
2 They decide on the objectives of the evaluation.
3 A group is elected to plan and organize the evaluation
4 The methods are chosen.
5 A written evaluation plan is developed.
6 Methods are prepared and tested.
7 Methods are used to collect information.
8 Information is analysed by participants – usually mainly by coordinators.
9 Results are reported in written, oral and visual form.
10 Programme participants decide how the results will be used.

In this process, the evaluation methods are chosen by a coalition of community and health organization and researcher partners. In practice, the research experts in the team suggest and guide the choice of methods. And these are often along the lines suggested by Butterfoss, above. Cornish (2006) has suggested that assessing participation in terms of 'more or less' does not adequately conceptualize what we mean by participation, and does not include the different forms of empowerment needed for different activities. Cornish conceptualizes participation in terms of concrete domains of action in which the participants may be empowered to act. To develop this conceptualization, she conducted a case study of participation by Indian sex workers in HIV prevention. The participants' activities were observed and analysed using ethnographic methods to study participation in the successful Sonagachi project (described in Chapter 7). Four different domains of participatory activity identified in this context were: accessing project services (e.g., accessing support); providing project services (e.g., health promotion work); shaping project workers' activity (e.g., participating in meetings); and participating in defining project goals (e.g., arguing for or against a particular organizational goal). A different set of resources is required for participation in each domain. Cornish argues that the domains of action, although they may appear to be in increasingly sophisticated levels of participation, are not hierarchical but qualitatively different and require quite different kinds of capacity. Thus, she suggests that evaluators must ask the question: 'Empowered to participate in what?' to consider the practical nature of different participatory activities.

Models for evaluating complex partnerships

Estable et al. (2006) grappled with participatory evaluation of a community-based health promotion project in some depth. In doing so they have drawn on and compared the use of a set of models for use in this challenging task. The *Mujer Sana/Communidad Sana* (Healthy Women/Healthy Communities) project aimed to increase the capacity of women in the Hispanic community in Ottawa, Canada, to participate in their own preventive health care. The project involved training members from this minority immigrant population to work with women in their communities as 'lay health promoters'. Four core partners were involved in developing the project for over three years (while other community members participated as advisers). The partners were: a Latin American women's group with strong networks in the community; a community health centre providing primary care and health promotion in an Ottawa neighbourhood; a small multilingual and multi-ethnic community-based consulting group, and a community health research unit based in the University of Ottawa and Ottawa Public Health. The project was conceived within a participatory action research framework using a lay health promotion model, and used participatory methods for ongoing evaluative feedback. 'The partners paid particular attention to ensuring that participation was not hindered by language differences, unequal economic resources, styles of working in meetings, organizational structures and constraints or different understandings about bureaucracy and community' (p. 32).

An original evaluation plan included process evaluation to be conducted by all members of the project team including the lay health promoters. The

Community Capacity Building Model (Moyer et al., 1999) was used to provide a framework for evaluation. The indicators used included type of community groups involved; the number of meetings attended; the diversity of organizations participating; the degree of commitment; readiness of organizations to work together; and sustainability of working relationships. In regard to power issues, the indicators included the empowerment of minority participants; the acceptance and integration of the minority community in the service delivery; the transferability of the lay health promotion model to other minority communities; and the removal of barriers to service access. The evaluation showed that the project had surpassed the original objectives. However, Estable et al. (2006) questioned whether this evaluation captured what had been learned about the partnership between groups with different resources, social status and ideals, during the project. To answer questions about levels of participation and changes in relationships that had not been addressed successfully by the indicators used, these authors applied three different frameworks to a *post hoc* evaluation of the complexities of partnership itself. These were the community capacity building model; Royal Society of Canada Guidelines for Appraising Participatory Research; and Key Moment Partnership Analysis.

The community capacity building model had also been applied to the original evaluation as a model for participatory process evaluation. The methods used were interviews with the partners, a document review and meeting notes. This model was useful in identifying the stages achieved in partnership development across time and recognizing the community leaders as key change agents. However, because this project had been initiated by the minority community rather than a public health practitioner, the processes did not always fit the model's stages.

The Royal Society of Canada Guidelines required each partner to complete a project participation self-assessment guide. This information was analysed to identify high and low consensus areas which was useful information for the evaluation. The data also provided a snapshot of each partner's understanding of participatory research. However, this model did not include a framework to explain why the differences found exist. Another limitation noted by the researchers was that this approach requires consensus on the terminology as used in the guidelines.

The Key Moment Partnership analysis was based on indications and gaps highlighted by application of the first two models. The authors used partnership indicators from the literature, an analysis of project documents and interviews with members of the partner organizations to review the development of the project. During this analysis, certain events and times became apparent as critical to the evaluation of partnership and these were called 'key moments'. Ten key moments were identified. They showed that the partnership itself had changed in important ways, such as making unexpected power dynamics visible, through the participatory evaluation. The complexity of this evaluation approach made it more difficult for all partners to participate and raised additional questions. In this project the authors acknowledge that participatory processes often burden those partners with the least resources in several ways. Nevertheless, the authors point to the positive outcomes of the participatory process in terms of gains in recognition for the minority partners and ongoing supportive relationships between the partners. The reflexive experiences of Estable et al. are valuable in considering the usefulness and limitations of various models and, more importantly, the complex issues involved in participatory practice including evaluation.

Issues in participatory evaluation

Participation has been recognized in public health practice as one of those words that are used to signify an unqualified good and lend a sense of legitimacy to a project. Many critics have pointed to the ways in which such buzz words may be used to cover many different types of practice, and to mask the problems and potentially harmful practices of intervention in any area. The friendly and positive sound of a word like 'participation' does not mean that we should abandon reflexive critique of its application. Springett (2003) has discussed a range of issues in participatory evaluation. Some of these, such as the need to balance the demands of participation against any benefits, the variation across contexts and the need for conceptual frameworks and appropriate tools have already been raised in the examples above. Many other important issues that she raises, such as tension between control by funders and community aims and timetables or struggles over the different agendas that are being brought together, are fundamentally about power relations. Naturally, when there are conflicting aims, agendas, needs and priorities, those with the most power provided by social class, social status, education and access to resources will tend to prevail. The inequalities in society are simply reflected in such relationships. Knowing this, it is incumbent on those in the most powerful positions to work toward the best use of their power and resources and to constantly reflect on the effects of their activities.

Power relations in community interventions

Wallerstein and Duran (2003) describe critiques of participatory studies in which the power relations are unexamined and their effects ignored. The importance of social relations in communities including those of gender, ethnicity, social class and age, or between researchers and community members, or funders and beneficiaries must be taken into account. Ignoring power imbalances in community empowerment initiatives can be extremely detrimental (Mukherjea, 2006). Recent evaluation research has included closer examination of the effects of these relationships on health promotion activities. This sort of research has been useful in explaining the problematic outcomes of many interventions and pointing towards a focus on understanding social relations and the socially embedded practices of everyday life as the very basis of health promotion process.

Following Cornish's (2006) study of participation and empowerment described above, Cornish and Ghosh (2007) turned to a study of power relations. They used the same ethnographic methods of observation of project activities and interviews with sex workers, development professionals, brothel managers and clients to examine how the Sonagachi Project has engaged with the inherently unequal social relations in the local context. Like many other health promotion projects of this nature, this project engaged with a community of participants (sex workers) who had very little social status and depended on others with more power (such as brothel keepers, clients or external project workers) for their living. Cornish and Ghosh's analysis of this situation showed that these more powerful interest groups were important forces in the project's development. It was necessary for the project organizers to accommodate the interests of local men's clubs and brothel managers. The economic and organizational capacity to run such a project has depended upon the direct input of development professionals and funding agencies. Thus, the project leaders are not the community of sex workers alone, but sex workers who are embedded in a social world with many powerful groups and complex interests that have had to be accommodated. For example, 'had the Project Director not occupied an authoritative role (in order to counter the power of sex workers' adversaries), and had the Project not negotiated carefully with club members and madams, it would not have survived and succeeded for 14 years' (p. 504). The engagement with these other groups was essential to the project's success, especially in the early stages. This success has led in turn to growing empowerment, prominence and respect for the sex workers as leaders. Cornish and Ghosh argue that a naive view of participation tends to sideline these important relations and to focus only on participation by the disadvantaged members. Rather than denying the existence of troubling power relations, it would be more useful to discuss and show how projects should be expected to plan for and include them.

Power relations in and beyond the community

Cornish and Ghosh focused on the role of local power relations and the importance of taking account of these forces in developing participation and empowerment for disadvantaged groups. Campbell (2003) has cast the net more widely to consider the ways in which community level interventions are embedded in local and society-wide power relations. While local social relations construct identities and behaviours, communities are also structured by the broader economic and social relations of wider society. As Mabala (2006) has pointed out, in the case of HIV/AIDS in particular, these include global relations. Campbell conducted a three-year process evaluation of a community HIV/AIDS prevention programme in South Africa (outlined in Chapter 7). The evaluation methods were ongoing in-depth interviews with residents, project workers and stakeholders, and an analysis of project documentation including policy documents, minutes of monthly stakeholder meetings and consultancy reports commissioned by the funding agencies. As the result of a complex and detailed analysis, Campbell describes the ways in which local power imbalances, such as those between men and women (sexual politics being particularly important in HIV/AIDS), tribal chiefs and their constituents, town dwellers and project organizers, and industrial stakeholders and project organizers, affected the project's conduct. For example, the multistakeholder partnerships (between the initiating group, mine management, trade unions, provincial and national government, and several researchers and international funding agencies) were riven with conflicts and imbalances, which Campbell teases out. She describes the effects of lack of political will in the country and region, and the lack of commitment to the aims of the project by powerful stakeholders such as the mining industry representatives. Leaders in industry and education joined the project while remaining committed to practices aimed at only changing individual behaviour among the town's people. They failed to take responsibility for their own role in potential change. Campbell argues that such prevention programmes must cultivate relation-ships between groups in society, not just within them, and must account for the social forces that are reproducing inequalities and ill health. In conclu-sion, she argues that:

> . . . the Summertown Project illustrates the immense complexities of implementing community-based HIV-prevention projects in the absence of an appropriate conceptualization of the interlocking bio-logical, psychological and social dimension of the epidemic, the devel-opment of local skills, capacity and infrastructure to translate such a vision into action, and the development of clear and robust incentives for effective stakeholder participation.
>
> (p. 186)

Power relations embedded in social institutions: the case of biomedicine

Campbell also notes that stakeholder groups may be dominated by bio-medically oriented doctors, nurses and researchers who '. . . do not auto-matically have the training or experience to manage complex projects' (p. 180). In health related projects, the biomedical approach, which incorpo-rates strong notions of hierarchy, high status for medically trained personnel and top–down expertise, is often the basis of tensions in participatory pro-jects based on ideals of empowerment and bottom–up ways of working. Springett (2003) mentions the detrimental influence of medical hegemony in developing participation in health related areas. This influence has been observed recently in evaluations of community projects. For example, Guareschi and Jovchelovitch (2004) have noted some of the challenging issues in a participatory project in Brazil designed to reduce inequalities by incorporating the demands of the poor into health policies. One of these is the consolidation of the power and status of medical professionals, which restricts participation of local community members in health teams. This reinforcement comes from both the professionals themselves (who prioritize medical knowledge) and from the community members (who fear the loss of medical services). Campbell et al. (2007) describe an example of the detrimental effects of this embedded power imbalance in a community development setting in Australia. A community development project in a remote Aboriginal community (see Chapter 7) was undermined and progress delayed owing to the reluctance of non-Aboriginal medical clinic staff to share control of health decisions with Aboriginal participants. Although the project was conceived as 'community driven', when the local people suggested different goals (broad child development needs rather than physical growth issues) and different solutions (a family centre for education and support), it became clear that the issues, solutions and implementation decisions were being driven by medical concerns and chosen by health professionals on the project team, and that they were unwilling to relinquish control. The health professionals resisted the needs expressed by the community and hampered the development of the centre. Although the group of Aboriginal community members succeeded in implementing their strategy, the community development process was much delayed and few initial health effects observed as outcomes based on the medical health criteria. The Aboriginal committee gained increased control of a community-based strategy, but did not succeed in influencing child health delivery services. 'Thus, while there were changes in power at the micro-level, the structures that limit the control Aboriginal community members have over their health services were not challenged' (p. 162). The Aboriginal people in Australia are already in an extremely unequal position, socially, economically and health-wise. Owing to the inequalities that are embedded in the health system itself, Campbell et al. question the capacity of government departments to practice community development. Such critiques based on process evaluations may not have immediate results in terms of well embedded institutional relationships and practices. Nevertheless, they are an important contribution to incremental changes in the ongoing development of health promotion activities.

Summary

Formative, process and outcome evaluation

This chapter has been structured around the evaluation of three aspects of intervention activities that have been well recognized in the literature: formative; process; and outcome evaluation. It is helpful to focus on these aspects as requiring different kinds of evaluation practices, but it is also important to recognize the blurring of boundaries between the three aspects. The evaluation of formative practices has important implications for processes and outcomes, and processes and outcomes themselves are inter-related in complex ways. In this chapter, I have also attempted to highlight the shifts across the meanings and values attached to these different stages of a health promotion intervention. The ways in which we understand the processes and how they relate to health outcomes depends on our theoretical perspective.

Glasgow and Emmons (2007) have noted these shifts and the ways in which the types of evidence required to evaluate health promotion activities are changing. In considering what types of evidence are needed, these authors critique the results of controlled trials and point to the importance of 'external validity' as an issue. In other words, context and process issues are an important part of outcomes. They suggest that multiple types of evidence and multiple outcomes should be considered and that these should allow for adaptation and refinement to suit local contexts.

Multiple methods

Several authors cited in this chapter and many others have suggested that the use of multiple research methods will assist the development of understanding about what actually happened during a health promotion programme, and what the outcomes are in relation to programme events and the local context. Approaches and methods that are appropriate to complex community-based health promotion programmes have been developed (e.g., Patton, 1997), and others recommend the use of qualtitative and quantitative methods to answer different research questions within an evaluation. These research questions should be based on the aims and theoretical basis of the programme and the methods chosen to be in accord with these.

Values

The desired processes and outcomes at any stage of a programme are not scientifically determined. They depend upon the values of those people who are guiding the intervention; and who those people are will depend in turn on the values underpinning the intervention. For example, a health promotion programme driven by health researchers and clinicians will value outcomes based on medical and scientific beliefs, whereas a programme developed in partnership with community members will value community chosen outcomes. Whether the values are those of science, humanism or local culture, recognizing the underlying values of our approach to programme development is an important aspect of a reflexive approach to health promotion. Likewise, a reflexive approach will help us to recognize and consider (if not always to solve immediately) the issues raised by conflicting values as health professionals and community members work together.

Evaluation as an iterative process

The basic purpose of evaluation activities should be to provide opportunities to improve or abandon certain practices and to point to useful directions for future development. The opportunity for reflection and suggestions provided for future improvements applies to all of the examples that have been discussed in this chapter, including those that employ experimental trials or those based on qualitative examination of process. For example, Campbell (2003) has written her book about a detailed process evaluation of the Summertown project with the aim of providing useful insights for future programme planners in the area of community-led HIV prevention and to contribute to consideration of increasing success. Visser et al. (2004) note that in this area, owing to the urgent importance of HIV/AIDS prevention, AIDS educators are actively building knowledge while implementing and evaluating programmes. They also suggest that it is through the detailed examination of obstacles and problems in current attempts that knowledge will be built for future projects.

In addition to such knowledge generated for the development of future health promotion work, evaluation of a particular programme may be used to develop that same programme in an ongoing way. This iterative approach to evaluation and practice is particularly appropriate within participatory interventions in which the goals and methods must be negotiated and developed in partnerships, and evaluation becomes an integral part of the ongoing processes of the programme. Community participatory projects are often based on the principles of action research. From this perspective, evaluation is not seen as some additional optional extra. It is conceptualized as an integral aspect of the process of development through iterative stages of health promotion practice.

Further reading

1 From a recognized leader in qualitative evaluation methods, this book includes sections on conceptual issues and theoretical orientations in qualitative inquiry with discussion of application to social action research. The book also provides descriptions of practical approaches including qualitative designs, methods and data collection, analysis, interpretation and reporting:

Patton, M.Q. (2002) *Qualitative Research & Evaluation Methods*, 3rd edn. Thousand Oaks, CA: Sage Publications.

2 An edited collection that brings together major evaluation researchers from a variety of social and behavioural science disciplines. Each chapter considers an issue in terms of implications for theory, method, practice or the profession, and explores approaches to dealing with the issue. Topics addressed include building evidence, cultural competence, involving stakeholders and synthesizing evaluation research findings:

Smith, N.L. and Brandon, P.R. (eds) (2007) *Fundamental Issues in Evaluation*. New York: Guilford Press.

3 A basic practical introduction to designing, conducting and analysing an evaluation study in healthcare. This book includes casestudies as examples and an introduction to developing methods and analysis skills:

Brophy, S., Snooks, H. and Griffiths, L. (2008) *Small-scale Evaluation in Health: A Practical Guide*. Thousand Oaks, CA: Sage Publications.

4 This book provides a practical and accessible approach to evaluation based on social service research and practice in the UK:

Everitt, A. and Hardiker, P. (1996) *Evaluating for Good Practice*. Houndmills, Basingstoke: Macmillan.

5 A book which presents ten principles of empowerment evaluation and describes tools for putting the principles into practice. Case study examples of diverse projects are provided which include community health foundation initiatives:

Fetterman, D.M. and Wandersman, A. (2004) *Empowerment Evaluation Principles in Practice*. New York: Guilford Press.

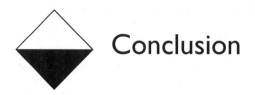 Conclusion

As we broaden the possibilities for psychological practice it may seem that the basis of that practice is no longer so clear cut. The range of choices for practical action may be confusing and seem difficult to assign to appropriate places. In broadening the basis of our understanding of individual behaviour and health to include the many levels of social life, and the recognition that these levels are enmeshed with the very basis of individual being, we are in danger of describing a universe that is too large to touch in any practical way. Reading about practices across all these levels within one book may make one feel this way. However, the purpose of this book is not to suggest that one should swallow the content whole and walk away into application. The purposes may be better described in terms of broadening options for application, suggesting a value-based reflexive approach to practice.

Thus, the first purpose is to suggest possibilities that will reverberate and suggest ways into further possibilities when we are working in particular situations. Health promoters will find themselves in all sorts of different practical situations depending on circumstances, but wherever one practises, access to a range of ideas and approaches can help. An example may help to explain what I mean here. A group of university-based community health promotion researchers recently began a project in a lower socioeconomic area, funded by government grants, to promote healthy eating and exercise. As these young researchers worked with the members of the community they found that they were talking to people who were keen to participate, keen to begin their own self-help groups, and brimming with ideas and enthusiasm about what their own health issues and health needs were, and what could be done about them. These researchers could see intuitively that this enthusiasm was being wasted by the way the current project was set up, but in actually carrying out the project activities and reporting to the wider community of psychologists, they were constrained by two factors: their own solid training in one traditional psychological approach to health promotion (which suggests that the government prescriptions for good health are the only truth and that they are the experts who know how people should behave), and the views of the medical experts who were also part of the project (that the community members are incapable of running their own groups). As these researchers describe the development of their project to the wider research community they feel somewhat schizoid. As members of the same social world they understand, relate to and can talk about the views of the people they are working with, but as scientists they must use another language to develop their interventions and report on their progress and research findings. With access to broader knowledge of what is 'legitimate' and 'allowed' to be discussed and practised by social scientists, this feeling of a divided self may be converted to one of an engaged and motivated practitioner.

The second and related broad purpose of the book is to emphasize ethical practice as an up front issue. Psychologists are very careful about ethical practice and very well trained to consider issues such as cultural sensitivity, confidentiality, informed consent, sexual attraction and competence to practice. In addition to these practical ethics, a community approach to health psychology suggests that the practitioner's values are in the foreground, and that values are the important basis of all choices across health issues, theory, research methods, interventions and evaluation. Considering values in this way leads the practitioner to consider the effect of their personal values on their practice, the values of all other participants and the values underlying the range of choices to be made. Many commentators in this area suggest that values should be the primary focus of evaluating the aims of health promotion rather than an instrumental or strategic focus. A move towards these sorts of aims opens the way for a more reflexive practice. A practitioner who is more aware of the different values implicated in different approaches, aware of the theoretical basis of their understandings of health and aware of the different values involved in different approaches to knowledge is in a position to make choices on this basis. Reflexive practice equips a health promoter to evaluate any number of models suggested for practice, either now or in the future.

Of course, the practice of health promotion will continue to evolve and change. Just as the new approaches that were being developed in health psychology only ten years ago are now passing their zenith, so, some of the more radical models described in this book will have soon have been trialled, found wanting and be out of favour. Nevertheless, now seems to be a good time to move in the direction pointed to by a social approach to understanding health. Positive ways to evolve should be based on developing our abilities to exchange knowledge and understandings of human well being with other disciplines, and directing our joint efforts toward health for all.

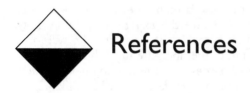

References

Abraham, C., Henderson, M. and Der, G. (2004) Cognitive impact of a research-based school sex education programme, *Psychology and Health*, 19(6), 689–703.

Abraham, C., Sheeran, P. and Wight, D. (1998) Designing research-based materials to promote safer sex amongst young people, *Psychology, Health and Medicine*, 3(1), 127–31.

Acheson, D. (1998) *Independent Inquiry into Inequalities in Health*. London: HMSO.

Adams, J., Witten, K. and Conway, K. (2007) Community development as health promotion: evaluating a complex locality-based project in New Zealand, *Community Development Journal*, DOI 10.1093/cdj/bsm049, 16 Nov.

Adler, N. (2006) When one's main effect is another's error: material vs. psychosocial explanations of health disparities. A commentary on Macleod et al., 'Is subjective social status a more important determinant of health than objective social status? Evidence from a prospective observational study of Scottish men', *Social Science and Medicine*, 63(4), 846–50.

African Union (2007) *Africa Health Strategy: 2007–2015. Third Session of the African Union Conference of Ministers of Health, Johannesburg, South Africa, 9–13 April, 2007*. Addis Ababa Ethiopia: African Union. Available at: www.africa-union.org/root/UA/Conferences/2007/avril/SA/9–13%20avr/doc/en/SA/AFRICA_HEALTH_STRATEGY_FINAL.doc (accessed 1 May 2007).

Annandale, E. and Hunt, K. (2000) Gender inequalities in health: research at the crossroads, in E. Annandale and K. Hunt (eds), *Gender Inequalities in Health*. Buckingham: Open University Press, pp. 1–35.

Annett, H. and Rifkin, S.B. (1995) *Guidelines for Rapid Participatory Appraisals to Assess Community Health Needs: A Focus on Health Improvements for Low Income Urban and Rural Areas*. Geneva: World Health Organization

Antonovsky, A. (1996) The salutogenic model as a theory to guide health promotion, *Health Promotion International*, 11(1), 11–18.

Arnstein, S.R. (1971) Eight rungs on the ladder of participation, in E.S. Cahn and B.A. Passett (eds), *Citizen Participation: Effecting Community Change*. New York: Praeger, pp. 69–91.

Artazcoz, L.L., Borrell, C., Benach, J., Cortès, I. and Rohlfs, I. (2004) Women, family demands and health: The importance of employment status and socio-economic position, *Social Science & Medicine*, 59(2), 263–74.

Assai, M., Siddiqi, S. and Watts, S. (2006) Tackling social determinants of health through community based initiatives, *British Medical Journal*, 333(7573), 854–6.

Bandura, A. (1977) Self-efficacy: toward a unifying theory of behavioral change. *Psychological Review*, 84(2), 191–215.

Bandura, A. (1986) *Social Foundations of Thought and Action: A Social Cognitive Theory*. Englewood Cliffs, NJ: Prentice-Hall.

Barnes, B.R. (2007) The politics of behavioural change for environmental health promotion in developing countries, *Journal of Health Psychology*, 12(3), 531–8.

Barnett, R., Pearce, J., and Moon, G. (2005) Does social inequality matter? Changing ethnic socio-economic disparities and Māori smoking in New Zealand, 1981–1996, *Social Science & Medicine*, 60(7), 1515–26.

Barreto, M.L. (2004) The globalization of epidemiology: critical thoughts from Latin America, *International Journal of Epidemiology*, 33(5), 1132–7.

Baum, F. (1999) Social capital: Is it good for your health? Issues for a public health agenda. *Journal of Epidemiology & Community Health*, 53, 195–6.

Beauchamp, D.E. (2003) Public health as social justice, in R. Hofrichter (ed.), *Health and Social Justice: Politics, Ideology, and Inequity in the Distribution of Disease*. San Francisco, CA: Jossey-Bass, pp. 267–84.

Becker, M.H. (1993) A medical sociologist looks at health promotion, *Journal of Health and Social Behaviour*, 34(1), 1–6.

Bennett, P. and Murphy, S. (1997) *Psychology and Health Promotion*. Buckingham: Open University Press.

Berkman, L.F., Glass, T., Brissette, I. and Seeman, T.E. (2000) From social integration to health: Durkheim in the new millennium, *Social Science & Medicine*, 51(6), 843–57.

Blakely, T. and Ivory, V. (2006) Commentary: bonding, bridging, and linking – but still not much going on, *International Journal of Epidemiology*, 35(3), 614–15.

Blakely, T., Fawcett, J., Hunt, D. and Wilson, N. (2006) What is the contribution of smoking and socioeconomic position to ethnic inequalities in mortality in New Zealand? *Lancet*, 368(9529), 44–52.

Blakely, T., Hunt, D. and Woodward, A. (2004) Confounding by socioeconomic position remains after adjusting for neighbourhood deprivation: an example using smoking and mortality, *Journal of Epidemiology & Community Health*, 58(12), 1030–1.

Blakely, T., Tobias, M., Robson, B., Ajwani, S., Bonne, M. and Woodward, A. (2005) Widening ethnic mortality disparities in New Zealand 1981–99, *Social Science & Medicine*, 61(10), 2233–51.

Blaxter, M. (1993) Why do the victims blame themselves? in A. Radley (ed.), *Worlds of Illness: Biographical and Cultural Perspectives on Health and Disease*. London: Routledge, pp. 124–42.

Blaxter, M. and Paterson, E. (1982) *Mothers and Daughters: A Three Generational Study of Health Attitudes and Behaviour*. London: Heinemann Educational.

Bolam, B. and Chamberlain, K. (2003) Professionalization and reflexivity in critical health psychology practice, *Journal of Health Psychology*, 8(2), 215–18.

Borrell, C., Muntaner, C., Benach, J. and Artazcoz, L. (2004) Social class and self-reported health status among men and women: what is the role of work organisation, household material standards and household labour? *Social Science & Medicine*, 58(10), 1869–87.

Bourdieu, P. (1977) *Outline of a Theory of Practice*, trans. R. Nice. Cambridge: Cambridge University Press.

Bourdieu, P. (1984) *Distinction: A Social Critique of the Judgement of Taste*. London: Routledge.

Bourdieu, P. (1986) The forms of capital, in J.G. Richardson (ed.), *Handbook of Theory and Research for the Sociology of Education*. Westport, CT: Greenwood Press, pp. 241–58.

Bradley, B.S., Deighton, J. and Selby, J. (2004) The 'Voices' Project: capacity-building in community development for youth at risk, *Journal of Health Psychology*, 9(2), 197–212.

Brandstatter, V., Lengfelder, A. and Gollwitzer, P.M. (2001) Implementation intentions and efficient action initiation, *Journal of Personality and Social Psychology*, 81(5), 946–60.

Breheny, M. and Stephens, C. (2007) Irreconcilable differences: health professionals' constructions of adolescence and motherhood, *Social Science & Medicine*, 64, 112–24.

Brezinka, V. and Kittel, F. (1996) Psychosocial factors of coronary heart disease in women: a review, *Social Science & Medicine*, 42(10), 1351–65.

Bronfenbrenner, U. (1979) *The Ecology of Human Development: Experiments by Nature and Design*. Cambridge, MA: Harvard University Press.

Brophy, S., Snooks, H. and Griffiths, L. (2008) *Small-scale Evaluation in Health: A Practical Guide*. Thousand Oaks, CA: Sage.

Brownson, R.C., Haire-Joshu, D. and Luke, D.A. (2006) Shaping the context of health: a review of environmental and policy approaches in the prevention of chronic diseases, *Annual Review of Public Health*, 27, 341–70.

Bruner, J. (1990) *Acts of Meaning*. Cambridge, MA: Harvard University Press.

Bryson, L. and Mowbray, M. (1981) 'Community': the spray-on solution, *Australian Journal of Social Issues*, 16, 255–67.

Buchanan, D. (2006) Moral reasoning as a model for health promotion, *Social Science & Medicine*, 63(10), 2715–26.

Burton, P., Goodlad, R. and Croft, J. (2006) How would we know what works? Context and complexity in the evaluation of community involvement, *Evaluation*, 12(3), 294–312.

Bury, M. (1982) Chronic illness as biographical disruption, *Sociology of Health & Illness*, 4(2), 167–82.

Butterfoss, F.D. (2006) Process evaluation for community participation, *Annual Review of Public Health*, 27, 323–40.

Byrd, W.M. and Clayton, L.A. (2003) Racial and ethnic disparities in healthcare: a background and history, in B. Smedley, A.Y. Stith, and A.R. Nelson (eds), *Unequal Treatment: Confronting Racial and Ethnic Disparities in Health Care*. Washington, DC: The National Academies Press, pp. 455–527.

Campbell, C. (2003) *Letting Them Die: Why HIV/AIDS Prevention Programmes fail*. Bloomington, IN: The International African Institute.

Campbell, C. and Gillies, P. (2001) Conceptualizing 'social capital' for health promotion in small local communities: a micro-qualitative study, *Journal of Community & Applied Social Psychology*, 11(5), 329–46.

Campbell, C. and Jovchelovitch, S. (2000) Health, community and development:

towards a social psychology of participation, *Journal of Community & Applied Social Psychology*, 10(4), 255–70.

Campbell, C. and Murray, M. (2004) Community health psychology: promoting analysis and action for social change, *Journal of Health Psychology*, 9(2), 187–95.

Campbell, C., Cornish, F. and Mclean, C. (2004) Social capital, participation and the perpetuation of health inequalities: obstacles to African-Caribbean participation in 'partnerships' to improve mental health, *Ethnicity & Health*, 9(4), 313–35.

Campbell, D., Wunungmurra, P. and Nyomba, H. (2007) Starting where the people are: lessons on community development from a remote Aboriginal Australian setting, *Community Development Journal*, 42(2), 151–66.

Carpiano, R.M. (2006) Toward a neighborhood resource-based theory of social capital for health: can Bourdieu and sociology help? *Social Science & Medicine*, 62(1), 165–75.

Carroll, D. and Davey Smith, G. (1997) Health and socio-economic position: a commentary, *Journal of Health Psychology*, 2(3), 275–82.

Carroll, D., Davey Smith, G. and Bennett, P. (1996) Some observations on health and socioeconomic status, *Journal of Health Psychology*, 1, 23–39.

Carson, A.J., Chappell, N.L. and Knight, C.J. (2007) Promoting health and innovative health promotion practice through a community arts centre, *Health Promotion Practice*, 8, 366–74.

Castro, A. and Farmer, P. (2003) Infectious disease in Haiti – HIV/AIDS, tuberculosis and social inequalities, *EMBO Reports*, 4, S20–S23.

Chamberlain, K. (1997) Socio-economic health differentials: from structure to experience, *Journal of Health Psychology*, 2(3), 399–411.

Chamberlain, K. (1999) Using grounded theory in health psychology, in M.M.K. Chamberlain (ed.), *Qualitative Health Psychology: Theories and Methods*. London: Sage, pp. 183–201.

Chamberlain, K. (2000) Methodolatry and qualitative health research, *Journal of Health Psychology*, 5(3), 285–96.

Chamberlain, K. (2004) Qualitative research, reflexivity and context, in M. Murray (ed.), *Critical Health Psychology*. Basingstoke: Palgrave, pp. 121–36.

Chamberlain, K. and O'Neill, D. (1998) Understanding social class differences in health: a qualitative analysis of smokers' health beliefs, *Psychology & Health*, 13(6), 1105–19.

Chapman, R.R. and Berggren, J.R. (2005) Radical contextualization: contributions to an anthropology of racial/ethnic health disparities, *Health (London)*, 9(2), 145–67.

Chappell, N., Funk, L., Carson, A., MacKenzie, P. and Stanwick, R. (2005) Multi-level community health promotion: how can we make it work? *Community Development Journal*, 41(3), 352–66.

Chattopadhyay, S.S. (2005) Not helpless victims of fate, *Frontline*, 22(8). Available at: www.hinduonnet.com/fline/fl2208/stories/20050422000708200.htm (accessed 31 August 2007).

Cho, H. and Salmon, C.T. (2007) Unintended effects of health communication campaigns, *Journal of Communication*, 57(2), 293–317.

Communication Initiative, The (2004) *Sonagachi Project – India*. Available at: www.comminit.com/experiences/pds12004/experiences-466.html (accessed 4 Sept. 2007).

Conner, M. and Norman, P. (1998) Health behaviour, in D.W. Johnston and

M. Johnston (eds), *Comprehensive Clinical Psychology. Volume 8: Health Psychology.* Amsterdam: Elsevier, pp. 1–37.

Cook, K.E. (2005) Using critical ethnography to explore issues in health promotion, *Qualitative Health Research*, 15(1), 129–38.

Cooke, R., Sniehotta, F. and Schuz, B. (2007) Predicting binge-drinking behavior using an extended TPB: examining the impact of anticipated regret and descriptive norms, *Alcohol and Alcoholism*, 42(2), 84–91.

Cornish, F. (2004) Making 'context' concrete: a dialogical approach to the society-health relation, *Journal of Health Psychology*, 9(2), 281–94.

Cornish, F. (2006) Empowerment to participate: a case study of participation by Indian sex workers in HIV prevention, *Journal of Community & Applied Social Psychology*, 16, 301–15.

Cornish, F. and Ghosh, R. (2007) The necessary contradictions of 'community-led' health promotion: a case study of HIV prevention in an Indian red light district, *Social Science & Medicine*, 64(2), 496–507.

Couldry, N. (2003) *Media Rituals: A Critical Approach.* London: Routledge.

Crawford, R. (1980) Healthism and the medicalisation of everyday life, *International Journal of Health Services*, 10(3), 365–88.

Cromby, J. (2007) Toward a psychology of feeling, *International Journal of Critical Psychology*, 21, 94–118.

Crossley, M.L. (2000a) *Rethinking Health Psychology.* Buckingham: Open University Press.

Crossley, M. (2000b) Narrative psychology, trauma and the study of self/identity, *Theory and Psychology*, 10, 527–46.

Crossley, M.L. (2001) Rethinking psychological approaches towards health promotion, *Psychology & Health*, 16(2), 161–77.

Crossley, N. (2001) *The Social Body: Habit, Identity and Desire.* London: Sage.

Crossley, M.L. (2002) 'Could you please pass one of those health leaflets along?' Exploring health, morality and resistance through focus groups, *Social Science & Medicine*, 55(8), 1471–83.

Crossley, N. (2002) *Making Sense of Social Movements.* Buckingham: Open University Press.

Crossley, M.L. (2003) 'Would you consider yourself a healthy person?' Using focus groups to explore health as a moral phenomenon, *Journal of Health Psychology*, 8(5), 501–14.

Crossley, M.L. (2004) Making sense of 'barebacking': gay men's narratives, unsafe sex and the 'resistance habitus', *British Journal of Social Psychology*, 43(2), 225–44.

Crotty, M. (1998) *The Foundations of Social Research: Meaning and Perspective in the Research Process.* London: Sage.

Dahlgren, G. and Whitehead, M. (1991) *Policies and Strategies to Promote Equity in Health.* Copenhagen: Regional Office for Europe, World Health Organization.

Davey Smith, G. (ed.). (2003) *Health Inequalities: Lifecourse Approaches.* Bristol: Policy Press.

Davey Smith, G., Hart, C., Blane, D., Gillis, C. and Hawthorne, V. (1997) Lifetime socioeconomic position and mortality: prospective observational study, *British Medical Journal*, 314, 547–52.

Davey Smith, G., McCarron, P., Okasha, M. and McEwen, J. (2001) Social circumstances in childhood and cardiovascular disease mortality: prospective observational study of Glasgow University students, *Journal of Epidemiology and Community Health*, 55, 340–1.

Davis, P., Beaglehole, R. and Durie, M. (2000) Directions for public health in New Zealand in the new millennium, *New Zealand Public Health Report*, 7, 1–10.

Deaton, A. and Lubotsky, D. (2003) Mortality, inequality and race in American cities and states, *Social Science & Medicine*, 56(6), 1139–53.

De-Graft Aikins, A. (2004) Strengthening quality and continuity of diabetes care in rural Ghana: a critical social psychological approach, *Journal of Health Psychology*, 9(2), 295–309.

Denton, M., Prus, S. and Walters, V. (2004) Gender differences in health: a Canadian study of the psychosocial, structural and behavioural determinants of health, *Social Science & Medicine*, 58(12), 2585–600.

DoH (Department of Health) (2004) *Choosing Health: Making Health Choices Easier*. London: HMSO. Available at: www.mlanortheast.org.uk/documents/ ChoosingHealthExecSummary.pdf (accessed 7 May 2007).

Diabetes Prevention Program Research Group (2002) Reduction in the incidence of type 2 diabetes with lifestyle intervention or metformin, *New England Journal of Medicine*, 346(6), 393–403.

Dickerson, S.S. and Kemeny, M.E. (2005) Acute stressors and cortisol responses, *Psychological Bulletin*, 130, 355–91.

Dinham, A. (2005) Empowered or over-powered? The real experiences of local participation in the UK's New Deal for Communities, *Community Development Journal*, 40(3), 301–12.

Durie, M. (1998) *Whaiora: Māori Health Development*, 2nd edn. Auckland, NZ: Oxford University Press.

Durie, M. (1999) *Te Pae Mahutonga*: a model for Māori health promotion. Unpublished paper, School of Māori Studies, Massey University, Palmerston North, New Zealand.

Durie, M. (2004) Understanding health and illness: research at the interface between science and indigenous knowledge. A key note address, World Congress of Epidemiology, Montreal, 20 August 2002, *International Journal of Epidemiology*, 33(5), 1138–43.

Eakin, J., Robertson, A., Poland, B., Coburn, D. and Edwards, R. (1996) Towards a critical social science perspective on health promotion research, *Health Promotion International*, 11, 157–65.

Earl, M. and National Health Committee (2002) The lifecourse approach to health and health inequalities: international evidence and its relevance to New Zealand / Aotearoa. Paper presented at the New Zealand Public Health Association Annual Conference, Dunedin, New Zealand, June.

Eckersly, R., Dixon, J. and Douglas, B. (eds) (2001) *The Social Origins of Health and Well-Being*. Cambridge: Cambridge University Press.

Edmondson, R. (2003) Social capital: a strategy for enhancing health? *Social Science & Medicine*, 57, 1723–33.

Ellis, B.H., Kia-Keating, M., Yusuf, S.A., Lincoln, A. and Nur, A. (2007) Ethical research in refugee communities and the use of community participatory methods, *Transcultural Psychiatry*, 44, 459–81.

Engel, G.L. (1977) The need for a new medical model: a challenge for biomedicine, *Science*, 196, 129–36.

Estable, A., Mechthild, M., Torres, S. and MacLean, L. (2006) Challenges of partici-
patory evaluation with a community-based health promotion partnership: '*Mujer
Sana, Communidad Sana* – Healthy Women, Healthy Communities', *The Canadian
Journal of Program Evaluation*, 21(2), 25–57.

Everitt, A. and Hardiker, P. (1996) *Evaluating for Good Practice*. Houndmills, Basingstoke: Macmillan.

Exworthy, M., Bindman, A., Davies, H. and Washington, A.E. (2006) Evidence into
policy and practice: measuring the progress of U.S. and U.K. policies to tackle
disparities and inequalities in U.S. and U.K. health and health care, *The Milbank
Quarterly*, 84, 75–109.

Fairhurst, E. (2005) Theorizing growing and being older: connecting physical
health, well-being and public health, *Critical Public Health*, 15(1), 27–38.

Farmer, P. (1994) AIDS-talk and the constitution of cultural models, *Social Science &
Medicine*, 38(6), 801–9.

Farmer, P. (1999) *Infections and Inequalities: The Modern Plagues*. Berkeley, CA: University of California Press.

Farrant, W. (1994) Addressing the contradictions: health promotion and community
health action in the United Kingdom, *Critical Public Health*, 5, 519.

Fassin, D. (2003) Le capital social, de la sociologie à l'épidémiologie: analyse critique
d'une migration transdiciplinaire, *Revue d'epidémiologie et de santé publique*, 51(3),
403–12 (full text in English available at: www.e2med.com/resp).

Feachem, R.G.A. (2000) Poverty and inequity: a proper focus for the new century,
Bulletin of the World Health Organization, 78(1), 1–2.

Felix, H.C. (2007) The rise of the community-based participatory research initiative
at the national institute for environmental health sciences: an historical analysis
using the policy streams model, *Progress in Community Health Partnerships: Research,
Education, and Action*, 1(1), 31–9.

Fetterman, D.M. and Wandersman, A. (2004) *Empowerment Evaluation Principles in
Practice*. New York: Guilford Press.

Fine, B. (2001) *Social Capital Versus Social Theory: Political Economy and Social Science
at the Turn of the Millennium*. London: Routledge.

Flick, U. (2000) Qualitative inquiries into social representations of health, *Journal of
Health Psychology*, 5(3), 315–25.

Flick, U. (2003) Editorial. Health concepts in different contexts, *Journal of Health
Psychology*, 8(5), 483–4.

Flisher, A.J., Lund, C., Funk, M. et al. (2007) Mental health policy development
and implementation in four African countries, *Journal of Health Psychology*, 12(3),
505–16.

Foucault, M. (1976) *The Birth of the Clinic: An Archaeology of Medical Perception*.
London: Tavistock.

Freire, P. (1972) *Pedagogy of the Oppressed*, trans. M.B. Ramos. Harmondsworth,
Middlesex: Penguin.

Freire, P. (1973) *Education for Critical Consciousness*. New York: Seabury Press.

Fullagar, S. (2002) Governing the healthy body: discourses of leisure and lifestyle
within Australian health policy, *Health (London)*, 6(1), 69–84.

Geiger, H.J. (2003) Racial and ethnic disparities in diagnosis and treatment: a review
of the evidence and a consideration of causes, in B. Smedley, A.Y. Stith and A.R.
Nelson (eds), *Unequal Treatment: Confronting Racial and Ethnic Disparities in Health
Care*. Washington, DC: The National Academies Press, pp. 417–54.

Gerbner, G., Gross, L., Morgan, M. and Signorielli, N. (1994) Growing up with television: the cultivation perspective, in J. Bryant and D. Zillmann (eds), *Media Effects Advances in Theory and Research*. Hove: Lawrence Erlbaum Associates, pp. 17–41.

Gibbs, A. (2007) Book review: C. Campbell, *Letting Them Die*: why HIV/AIDS prevention programmes fail, *Journal of Health Psychology*, 12, 557–9.

Glanz, K., Rimer, B.K. and Lewis, F.M. (eds) (2002) *Health Behaviour and Health Education: Theory, Research, and Practice*, 3rd edn. San Francisco, CA: Jossey-Bass.

Glasgow, R.E. and Emmons, K.M. (2007) How can we increase translation of research into practice? Types of evidence needed, *Annual Review of Public Health*, 28, 413–33.

Glover, M. (2005) Analysing smoking using Te Whare Tapa Wha, *New Zealand Journal of Psychology*, 34(1), 13–19.

Goldstein, D.E. (2000) 'When ovaries retire': contrasting women's experiences with feminist and medical models of menopause, *Health (London)*, 4, 309–23.

Good, M.-J.D., James, C., Good, B.J. and Becker, A.E. (2003) The culture of medicine and racial, ethnic, and class disparities in healthcare, in B. Smedley, A.Y. Stith and A.R. Nelson (eds), *Unequal Treatment: Confronting Racial and Ethnic Disparities in Health Care*. Washington, DC: The National Academies Press, pp. 594–624.

Goodwin, I. (2003) Reconceptualising virtual community: a case study of Internet use in Birmingham. Unpublished PhD thesis, University of Birmingham, Birmingham.

Green, L.W., Poland, B.D. and Rootman, I. (2000) The settings approach to health promotion, in B.D. Poland, L.W. Green and I. Rootman (eds), *Settings for Health Promotion: Linking Theory and Practice*. Thousand Oaks: Sage, pp. 1–44.

Greenhalgh, T., Collard, A. and Begum, N. (2005a) Sharing stories: complex intervention for diabetes education in minority ethnic groups who do not speak English, *British Medical Journal*, 330(7492), 628–34.

Greenhalgh, T., Collard, A. and Begum, N. (2005b) Narrative based medicine, *Practical Diabetes International*, 22(4), 125–9.

Guareschi, P.A. and Jovchelovitch, S. (2004) Participation, health and the development of community resources in Southern Brazil, *Journal of Health Psychology*, 9(2), 311–22.

Guldan, G.S. (1996) Obstacles to community health promotion, *Social Science & Medicine*, 43(5), 689–95.

Guttman, N. (2000) *Public Health Communication Interventions: Values and Ethical Dilemmas*. Thousand Oaks, CA: Sage.

Habermas, J. (1984) *The Theory of Communicative Action: Reason and the Rationalization of Society (Volume 1)*, trans. T. McCarthy. Boston: Beacon Press.

Habermas, J. (1987) *The Theory of Communicative Action: Reason and the Rationalization of Society (Volume 2)*, trans. T. McCarthy. Cambridge: Polity Press.

Habermas, J. (1990) *Moral Consciousness and Communicative Action*, trans. C. Lenhardt and S.W. Nicholson. Cambridge, MA: MIT Press.

Hadera, H., Boer, H. and Kuiper, W. (2007) Using the theory of planned behaviour to understand the motivation to learn about HIV/AIDS prevention among adolescents in Tigray, Ethiopia, *AIDS Care*, 19(7), 895–900.

Haraway, D.J. (1991) *Simians, Cyborgs, and Women*. New York: Routledge.

Hardey, M. (1998) *The Social Context of Health*. Buckingham: Open University Press.

Harré, R. and Gillett, G. (1994) *The Discursive Mind*. London: Sage.

Harris, R., Tobias, M., Jeffrey, M. et al. (2006) Effects of self-reported racial discrimination and deprivation on Māori health and inequalities in New Zealand: cross-sectional study, *Lancet*, 367(9527), 2005–9.

Hastings, G. and McDermott, L. (2006) Putting social marketing into practice, *British Medical Journal*, 332, 1210–12.

Hawe, P. and Shiell, A. (2000) Social capital and health promotion: a review, *Social Science & Medicine*, 51(6), 871–85.

Heller, K., Price, R.H., Reinharz, S. et al. (1984) *Psychology and Community Change: Challenges of the Future*, 2nd edn. Homewood, IL: Dorsey Press.

Hepworth, J. (2004) Public health psychology: a conceptual and practical framework, *Journal of Health Psychology*, 9(1), 41–54.

Herzlich, C. (1973) *Health and Illness: A Social Psychological Analysis*. London: Academic Press.

Hillery, G.A. (1955) Definitions of community: areas of agreement, *Rural Sociology*, 20, 111–24.

Hisamichi, S. (2004) Science and ethics in epidemiology, *Journal of Epidemiology*, 14(4), 105–11.

Ho, L.S., Gittelsohn, J., Harris, S.B. and Ford, E. (2006) Development of an integrated diabetes prevention program with First Nations in Canada, *Health Promotion International*, 21(2), 88.

Hodgetts, D., Bolam, B. and Stephens, C. (2005) Mediation and the construction of contemporary understandings of health and lifestyle, *Journal of Health Psychology*, 10(1), 123–36.

Hofrichter, R. (2003) The politics of health inequities: contested terrain, in R. Hofrichter (ed.), *Health and Social Justice: Politics, Ideology, and Inequity in the Distribution of Disease*. San Francisco, CA: Jossey-Bass, pp. 1–56.

Howarth, C., Foster, J. and Dorrer, N. (2004) Exploring the potential of the theory of social representations in community-based health research – and vice versa? *Journal of Health Psychology*, 9(2), 229–43.

Howden-Chapman, P., Matheson, A., Crane, J. et al. (2007) Effect of insulating existing houses on health inequality: cluster randomised study in the community, *British Medical Journal* (doi:10.1136/bmj.39070.573032.573080), 334, 460.

Human Rights and Equal Opportunity Commission (2008) Indigenous health campaign. Available at: www.hreoc.gov.au/social_justice/health/index.html (accessed 11 Feb. 2008).

Humpage, L. (2006) An 'inclusive' society: a 'leap forward' for Māori in New Zealand? *Critical Social Policy*, 26(1), 220–42.

Hunter, D.J. (2005) Choosing or losing health? *Journal of Epidemiology and Community Health*, 59(12), 1010–13.

Illich, I. (1977) *Limits to Medicine: Medical Nemesis. The Expropriation of Health*. Harmondsworth: Penguin.

Jackson, C., Lawton, R., Knapp, P. et al. (2005) Beyond intention: do specific plans increase health behaviours in patients in primary care? A study of fruit and vegetable consumption, *Social Science & Medicine*, 60(10), 2383–91.

Jamieson, L.M., Parker, E.J. and Armfield, J.M. (2007) Indigenous child oral health at a regional and state level, *Journal of Paediatrics and Child Health*, 43(3), 117–21.

Jana, S., Bandyopadhyay, N., Saha, A. and Dutta, M.K. (1999) Creating an enabling environment: lessons learnt from the Sonagachi Project, India, *Research for Sex*

Work, 2. Available at: http://hcc.med.vu.nl/artikelen/jana.htm (accessed 31 Aug. 2007).

Jana, S., Basu, I., Rotheram-Borus, M.J. and Newman, P.A. (2004) The Sonagachi project: a sustainable community intervention program, *AIDS Education and Prevention*, 16(5), 405–14.

Jemmott, J., Heeren, G., Ngwane, Z. et al. (2007) Theory of planned behavior predictors of intention to use condoms among Xhosa adolescents in South Africa, *AIDS Care*, 19(5), 677–84.

Jodelet, D. (1991) *Madness and Social Representations: Living with the Mad in One French Community*, trans. T. Pownall. Berkeley, CA: University of California Press.

Joffe, H. and Bettega, N. (2003) Social representation of AIDS among Zambian adolescents, *Journal of Health Psychology*, 8(5), 616–31.

Joffe, H. and Lee, N.Y.L. (2004) Social representation of a food risk: the Hong Kong avian bird flu epidemic, *Journal of Health Psychology*, 9(4), 517–33.

Kahl, M.L. and Lawrence-Bauer, J. (1996) An analysis of discourse promoting mammography: pain, promise, and prevention, in R.L. Parrott and M.C. Condit (eds), *Evaluating Women's Health Messages*. Thousand Oaks, CA: Sage, pp. 307–25.

Kaplan, G.A., Pamuk, E.R., Lynch, J.W., Cohen, R.D. and Balfour, J.L. (1996) Inequality in income and mortality in the United States: analysis of mortality and potential pathways, *British Medical Journal*, 312(7037), 999–1003.

Kawachi, I., Kennedy, B.P., Lochner, K. and Prothrow-Stith, D. (1997) Social capital, income inequality, and mortality, *American Journal of Public Health*, 87(9), 1491–8.

Kemmis, S. and McTaggart, R. (2000) Participatory action research, in N.K. Denzin and Y.S. Lincoln (eds), *Handbook of Qualitative Research*. Thousand Oaks, CA: Sage, pp. 567–607.

Kemp, L., Chavez, R., Harris-Roxas, B. and Burton, N. (2007) What's in the box? Issues in evaluating interventions to develop strong and open communities, *Community Development Journal*, Advance Access (DOI 10.1093/cdj/bsm014), 5 June.

Khanlou, N. and Peter, E. (2005) Participatory action research: considerations for ethical review, *Social Science & Medicine*, 60, 2333–40.

Kok, G., Hospers, H., Harterink, P. and de Zwart, O. (2007) Social-cognitive determinants of HIV risk-taking intentions among men who date men through the Internet, *AIDS Care*, 19(3), 410–17.

Kok, G., Schaalma, H., Ruiter, R.A.C., Van Empelen, P. and Brug, J. (2004) Intervention mapping: protocol for applying health psychology theory to prevention programmes, *Journal of Health Psychology*, 9(1), 85–98.

Krause, M. (2003) The transformation of social representations of chronic disease in a self-help group, *Journal of Health Psychology*, 8(5), 599–615.

Kros, S., Wong, M., Dy, B. et al. (2004) Exporting Kurt Lewin's (1946) action research to Cambodia: confronting the cultural, gender and disciplinary particularities of combating HIV/AIDS, *Australian Journal of Psychology*, 56(Supp. 1), 75.

Labonte, R. (2005) Editorial: towards a critical population health research, *Critical Public Health*, 15(1), 1–3.

Labonte, R. and Laverack, G. (2001) Capacity building in health promotion, Part 1: for whom? And for what purpose? *Critical Public Health*, 11(2), 111–27.

Labonte, R., Muhajarine, N., Abonyl, S. et al. (2002) An integrated exploration in the social and environmental determinants of health: the Saskatchewan Population Health and Evaluation Unit (SPHERU), *Chronic Diseases in Canada*, 23(2), 71–6.

Labonte, R., Polanyi, M., Muhajarine, N., McIntosh, T. and Williams, A. (2005) Beyond the divides: towards critical population health research, *Critical Public Health*, 15(1), 5–17.

Laverack, G. (2007) *Health Promotion Practice: Building Empowered Communities*. Maidenhead: Open University Press.

Levin, B.W. and Browner, C.H. (2005) The social production of health: critical contributions form evolutionary, biological, and cultural anthropology, *Social Science & Medicine*, 61, 745–50.

Levins, R. (2003) Is capitalism a disease? The crisis in U.S. public health, in R. Hofrichter (ed.), *Health and Social Justice: Politics, Ideology, and Inequity in the Distribution of Disease*. San Francisco, CA: Jossey-Bass, pp. 365–84.

Lewin, K. (1946) Action research and minority problems, *Journal of Social Issues*, 2, 34–46.

Lewin K. ([1948] 1997) *Resolving Social Conflicts and Field Theory in Social Science*. Washington, DC: American Psychological Association.

Liu, J.H. and Ng, S.H. (2007) Connecting Asians in global perspective: special issue on past contributions, current status and future prospects for Asian social psychology, *Asian Journal of Social Psychology*, 10(1), 1–7.

Liu, M., Gao, R. and Pusari, N. (2006) Using participatory action research to provide health promotion for disadvantaged elders in Shaanxi Province, China, *Public Health Nursing*, 23(4), 332–8.

Lubek, I. (2003) Book review: P. Farmer, *Infections and Inequalities: The Modern Plagues*, *Culture Health & Sexuality*, 5(2), 175–9.

Lubek, I., Wong, M.L., McCourt, M. et al. (2002) Collaboratively confronting the current Cambodian HIV/AIDS crisis in Siem Reap: a cross-disciplinary, cross-cultural 'participatory action research' project in consultative, community health change, *Asian Psychologist*, 3(1), 21–8.

Lubek, I., Wong, M.L., Dy, B.C. et al. (2003) Only 'beer girls', no 'beer boys' in Cambodia: confronting globalisation and inequalities in literacy, poverty, employment, and risk for HIV/AIDS, *Australian Journal of Psychology*, 55(Supp. 1), 51.

Lubek, I., Lee, H., Kros, S. et al. (2004) Lessons from social psychology: changing public opinion and corporate policies about HIV/AIDS in the developing world, *Australian Journal of Psychology*, 56(Supp. 1), 77.

Lubek, I., Schuster, J., Cadesky, J. et al. (2005) Health promotion vs. beer promotion in Cambodia and Canada: some comparative observations on the social context of social (ir)responsibility and social action responses, *Australian Journal of Psychology*, 57(Supp. 1), 94.

Lubek, I., Kros, S., Mu, S. et al. (2006) Beyond the social construction to the community construction of health: roles for applied social psychologists within a multi-sectoral confrontation of HIV/AIDS, alcohol abuse and violence against women in Siem Reap, Cambodia, *Australian Journal of Psychology*, 58(Supp. 1), 37.

Lupton, D. (1995) *The Imperative of Health: Public Health and the Regulated Body*. London: Sage.

Lykes, M.B. (2000) Possible contributions of a psychology of liberation: whither health and human rights? *Journal of Health Psychology*, 5(3), 383–97.

Lykes, M.B., Blanche, M.T. and Hamber, B. (2003) Narrating survival and change in Guatemala and South Africa: the politics of representation and a liberatory community psychology, *American Journal of Community Psychology*, 31(1–2), 79–90.

Lynch, J.W., Davey Smith, G., Kaplan, G. and House, J.S. (2000) Income inequality and mortality: importance to health of individual income, psychosocial environment, or material conditions, *British Medical Journal*, 320(29 Apr.), 1200–4.

Lynch, J., Due, P., Muntaner, C. and Davey Smith, G. (2000) Social capital – is it a good investment strategy for public health? *Journal of Epidemiology & Community Health*, 54(6), 404–8.

Lynch, J., Harper, S. and Davey Smith, G. (2003) Commentary: plugging leaks and repelling boarders – where to next for the SS Income Inequality? *International Journal of Epidemiology*, 32(6), 1029–36.

Lyons, A. (2000) Examining media representations: benefits for health psychology, *Journal of Health Psychology*, 5(3), 349–58.

Lyons, A. and Chamberlain, K. (2006) *Health Psychology: A Critical Introduction*. Cambridge: Cambridge University Press.

Mabala, R. (2006) From HIV prevention to HIV protection: addressing the vulnerability of girls and young women in urban areas, *International Institute for Environment and Development*, 18(2), 407–32.

Macaulay, A.C., Paradis, G., Potvin, L. et al. (1997) The Kahnawake schools diabetes prevention project: intervention, evaluation, and baseline results of a diabetes primary prevention program with a native community in Canada, *Preventive Medicine*, 26(6), 779–90.

Macinko, J. and Starfield, B. (2001) The utility of social capital in research on health determinants, *The Milbank Quarterly*, 79, 387–427.

MacIntyre, S. and Hunt, K. (1997) Socio-economic position, gender and health: how do they interact? *Journal of Health Psychology*, 2(3), 315–34.

Maclean, L.M., Diem, E., Bouchard, C. et al. (2007) Complexity and team dynamics in multiple intervention programmes: challenges and insights for public health psychology, *Journal of Health Psychology*, 12, 341–51.

Marks, D.F. (2004). Rights to health, freedom from illness: a life and death matter, in M. Murray (ed.), *Critical Health Psychology*. Basingstoke: Palgrave, pp. 61–82.

Marmot, M. (1999) Epidemiology of socioeconomic status and health: are determinants within countries the same as between countries? *Annals of the New York Academy of Sciences*, 896(1), 16–29.

Marmot, M. (2004a) Tackling health inequalities since the Acheson Inquiry, *Journal of Epidemiology & Community Health*, 58(4), 262–3.

Marmot, M. (2004b) *The Status Syndrome: How Social Standing Affects Our Health and Longevity*. New York: Henry Holt.

Marmot, M., and Smith, G.D. (1997) Socio-economic differentials in health, *Journal of Health Psychology*, 2(3), 283–96.

Marmot, M., Shipley, M.J. and Rose, G. (1984) Inequalities in death: specific explanations of a general pattern? *Lancet*, 1, 1003–6.

Marmot, M., Stansfeld, S., Patel, C. et al. (1991) Health inequalities among British civil servants: the Whitehall II study, *Lancet*, 337(8754), 1387–93.

Matheson, A., Howden-Chapman, P. and Dew, K. (2005) Engaging communities to reduce inequalities in health: why partnership? *Social Policy Journal of New Zealand*, 26, 1–16.

McCreanor, T. and Nairn, R. (2002) Tauiwi general practitioners' explanations of Māori health: colonial relations in primary healthcare in Aotearoa/New Zealand? *Journal of Health Psychology*, 7(5), 509–18.

McCreanor, T. and Watson, P. (2004) Resiliency, connectivity and environments:

their roles in theorising approaches to promoting the well-being of young people, *International Journal of Mental Health Promotion*, 6(1), 38–41.

McIntyre, A. (2007) *Participatory Action Research*. Thousand Oaks, CA: Sage.

McKeown, T. (1979) *The Role of Medicine: Dream, Mirage or Nemesis?* 2nd edn. Oxford: Basil Blackwell.

McLeroy, K.R., Norton, B.L., Kegler, M.C., Burdine, J.N. and Sumaya, C.V. (2003) Community-based interventions, *American Journal of Public Health*, 93(4), 529–33.

McMillan, B., Higgins, A.R. and Conner, M. (2005) Using an extended theory of planned behaviour to understand smoking amongst schoolchildren, *Addiction Research & Theory*, 13(3), 293–306.

Merzel, C. and D'Afflitti, J. (2003) Reconsidering community-based health promotion: promise, performance, and potential, *American Journal of Public Health*, 93(4), 557–74.

Ministry of Health, New Zealand (2000) *New Zealand Health Strategy*, December. Available at: www.moh.govt.nz/moh.nsf

Ministry of Health, New Zealand (2002) *Reducing Inequalities in Health*. Wellington, NZ: Ministry of Health. Available at: http://www.moh.govt.nz

Minkler, M. and Wallerstein, N. (eds) (2003) *Community-based Participatory Research for Health*. San Francisco, CA: Jossey-Bass.

Misra, R. and Ballard, D. (2003) Community needs and strengths assessment as an active learning project, *The Journal of School Health*, 73, 269–71.

Moore, S., Haines, V., Hawe, P. and Shiell, A. (2006) Lost in translation: a genealogy of the 'social capital' concept in public health, *Journal of Epidemiology and Community Health*, 60(8), 729–34.

Morgan, M. (1999) Discourse, health and illness, in M. Murray and K. Chamberlain (eds), *Qualitative Health Psychology: Theories and Methods*. London: Sage, pp. 64–82.

Morgan, L.M. (2001) Community participation in health: perpetual allure, persistent challenge, *Health Policy and Planning*, 16, 221–30.

Moscovici, S. and Duveen, G. (2000) *Social Representations: Explorations in Social Psychology*. Cambridge: Polity Press.

Moss, N.E. (2003) Socioeconomic disparities in health in the United States: an agenda for action, in R. Hofrichter (ed.), *Health and Social Justice: Politics, Ideology, and Inequity in the Distribution of Disease*. San Francisco, CA: Jossey-Bass, pp. 501–21.

Moyer, A., Coristine, M., MacLean, L. and Meyer, M. (1999) A model for building collective capacity in community-based programs: the Elderly in Need Project, *Public Health Nursing*, 16(3), 205–14.

Mueller, E.J. and Tighe, J.R. (2007) Making the case for affordable housing: connecting housing with health and education outcomes, *Journal of Planning Literature*, 21(4), 371–85.

Mukherjea, A. (2006) Conceptualizing and assessing community-based HIV prevention work: a case study in South Africa, *Health (London)*, 10(3), 369–74.

Muntaner, C., Lynch, J. and Davey Smith, G. (2001) Social capital, disorganized communities, and the third way: understanding the retreat from structural inequalities in epidemiology and public health, *International Journal of Health Services*, 31(2), 213–37.

Murphy, S. and Bennett, P. (2004) Health psychology and public health: theoretical possibilities, *Journal of Health Psychology*, 9(1), 13–27.

Murray, M. (2000) Levels of narrative analysis in health psychology, *Journal of Health Psychology*, 5(3), 337–47.

Murray, M. and Campbell, C. (2003) Living in a material world: reflecting assumptions of health psychology, *Journal of Health Psychology*, 8(2), 231–6.

Murray, M. and Chamberlain, K. (eds) (1999) *Qualitative Health Psychology: Theories and Methods*. London: Sage.

Murray, M. and Poland, B. (2006) Health psychology and social action, *Journal of Health Psychology*, 11(3), 379–84.

Murray, M. and Tilley, N. (2005) *The Bottom Line: Developing Safety Awareness in Fishing Communities Through Community Arts*. Newfoundland, Canada: SafetyNet, Memorial University of Newfoundland.

Murray, M. and Tilley, N. (2006) Promoting safety awareness in fishing communities through community arts: an action research project, *Safety Science*, 44(9), 797–808.

Murray, M., Pullman, D. and Rodgers, T.H. (2003) Social representations of health and illness among 'baby-boomers' in Eastern Canada, *Journal of Health Psychology*, 8(5), 485–99.

Murray, M., Nelson, G., Poland, B., Maticka-Tyndale, E. and Ferris, L. (2004) Assumptions and values of community health psychology, *Journal of Health Psychology*, 9(2), 323–33.

National Institute of Public Health Sweden (2003) *National Public Health Strategy for Sweden in Brief*. Available at: www.fhi.se/shop/material_pdf/strategy.pdf (accessed 1 May 2007).

Ndirangu, M., Perkins, H., Yadrick, K. et al. (2007) Conducting needs assessment using the comprehensive participatory planning and evaluation model to develop nutrition and physical activity interventions in a rural community in the Mississippi Delta, *Progress in Community Health Partnerships: Research, Education, and Action*, 1(1), 41–8.

Nelson, G. and Prilleltensky, I. (2005) *Community Psychology: In Pursuit of Liberation and Wellbeing*. New York: Palgrave Macmillan.

Nelson, G., Pancer, S.M., Hayward, K. and Kelly, R. (2004) Partnerships and participation of community residents in health promotion and prevention: experiences of the Highfield Community Enrichment Project (Better Beginnings, Better Futures), *Journal of Health Psychology*, 9(2), 213–27.

Nelson, G., Pancer, M., Hayward, K. and Peters, R.D. (2005) *Partnerships for Prevention: The Story of the Highfield Community Enrichment Project*. Toronto, ON: Toronto University Press.

Nguyen, V.M. and Peschard, K. (2003) Anthropology, inequality, and disease: a review, *Annual Review of Anthropology*, 32, 447–74.

Nightingale, D.J. and Cromby, J. (eds) (1993) *Social Constructionist Psychology: A Critical Analysis of Theory and Practice*. Buckingham: Open University Press.

Norris, S.L., Engelgau, M.M. and Venkat Narayan, K.M. (2001) Effectiveness of self-management training in type 2 diabetes: a systematic review of randomized controlled trials, *Diabetes Care*, 24(3), 561–87.

Nutbeam, D. (1998) Evaluating health promotion: progress, problems and solutions, *Health Promotion International*, 13, 27–44.

Ogden, J. (2004) *Health Psychology: A Text Book*, 3rd edn. Maidenhead: Open University Press.

Ohrling, S. (2003) *Sweden's National Public Health Strategy: Relating National Targets to*

Determinants Rather than Diseases or Illnesses. Stockholm: Swedish National Institute of Public Health. Available at: http://secure.cihi.ca/cihiweb/en/downloads/cphi_Ohrling_e.pdf (accessed 1 May 2007).

Owen, N., Humpel, N., Leslie, E., Bauman, A. and Sallis, J.F. (2004) Understanding environmental influences on walking: review and research agenda, *American Journal of Preventive Medicine*, 27(1), 67–76.

Pancer, S.M., Nelson, G., Dearing, B. et al. (2003) Highfield Community Enrichment Project (Better Beginnings, Better Futures): a community-based project for the promotion of wellness in children and families, in K. Kufeldt and B. McKenzie (eds), *Child Welfare: Connecting Research, Policy and Practice*. Waterloo, ON: Wilfrid Laurier University Press.

Parker, I. (2005) *Qualitative Psychology: Introducing Radical Research*. Maidenhead: Open University Press.

Patten, S., Mitton, C. and Donaldson, C. (2006) Using participatory action research to build a priority setting process in a Canadian Regional Health Authority, *Social Science & Medicine*, 63(5), 1121–34.

Patton, M.Q. (2002) *Qualitative Research & Evaluation Methods*, 3rd edn. Thousand Oaks, CA: Sage.

Paul, V. (2004) Health systems and the community, *British Medical Journal*, 329(7475), 1117–18.

Pearce, N. (2003) Which community? *Public Health Association (NZ) News*, 6(5), 3–4.

Pearce, N. (2004) The globalization of epidemiology: introductory remarks, *International Journal of Epidemiology*, 33(5), 1127–31.

Pearce, N. and Smith, G.D. (2003) Is social capital the key to inequalities in health? *American Journal of Public Health*, 93(1), 122–9.

Pepall, E., Earnest, J. and James, R. (2007) Understanding community perceptions of health and social needs in a rural Balinese village: results of a rapid participatory appraisal, *Health Promotion International*, 22(1), 44–52.

Pérez, D., Lefèvre, P., Sánchez, L. et al. (2007) Community participation in *Aedes aegypti* control: a sociological perspective on five years of research in the health area '26 de Julio', Havana, Cuba, *Tropical Medicine & International Health*, 12(5), 664–72.

Petersen, A. and Lupton, D. (1996) *The New Public Health: Health and Self in the Age of Risk*. London: Sage.

Poland, B. (1992) Learning to 'walk our talk': the implications of sociological theory for research methodologies in health promotion, *Canadian Journal of Public Health*, 83(S1), S31–S46.

Popay, J., Bartley, M. and Owen, C. (1993) Gender inequalities in health: social position, affective disorders and minor physical morbidity, *Social Science & Medicine*, 36(1), 21–32.

Popple, K. (1995) *Analysing Community Work: Its Theory and Practice*. Bristol, PA: Open University Press.

Porter, C. (2007) Ottawa to Bangkok: changing health promotion discourse, *Health Promotion International*, 22(1), 72–9.

Portes, A. (1998) Social capital: its origins and applications in modern sociology, *Annual Review of Sociology*, 24(1), 1–24.

Potter, J. and Wetherell, M. (1987) *Discourse and Social Psychology: From Attitudes to Behaviour*. London: Sage.

Potvin, L., Cargo, M., McComber, A.M., Delormier, T. and Macaulay, A.C. (2003) Implementing participatory intervention and research in communities: lessons from the Kahnawake Schools Diabetes Prevention Project in Canada, *Social Science & Medicine*, 56(6), 1295–305.

Prilleltensky, I. and Prillelltensky, O. (2003) Towards a critical health psychology practice, *Journal of Health Psychology*, 8(2), 197–210.

Pugh, H., Power, C., Goldblatt, P. and Arber, S. (1991) Women's lung cancer mortality, socio-economic status and changing smoking patterns, *Social Science & Medicine*, 32(10), 1105–10.

Putnam, R.D. (1995) Bowling alone: America's declining social capital, *Journal of Democracy*, 6, 65–78.

Putnam, R.D. (2004) Commentary: 'Health by association': some comments, *International Journal of Epidemiology*, 33(4), 667–71.

Putnam, R.D. and Feldstein, L.M. (2003) *Better Together: Restoring the American Community*. New York: Simon & Schuster.

Radley, A. (ed.) (1993) *Worlds of Illness: Biographical and Cultural Perspectives on Health and Disease*. London: Routledge.

Radley, A. (1994) *Making Sense of Illness: The Social Psychology of Health and Disease*. London: Sage.

Radley, A. (1997) What role does the body have in illness? in L. Yardley (ed.), *Material Discourses of Health and Illness*. Florence, KY: Taylor & Frances/Routledge, pp. 50–67.

Radley, A. (2003) Review of 'Phenomenology encounters illness: beyond inner states', *Health*, 7(2), 255–60.

Radley, A. and Billig, M. (1996) Accounts of health and illness: dilemmas and representations, *Sociology of Health & Illness*, 18(2), 220–40.

Raeburn, J., Akerman, M., Chuengsatiansup, K., Mejia, F. and Oladepo, O. (2006) Community capacity building and health promotion in a globalized world, *Health Promotion International*, 21(supp. 1), 84–90.

Ramella, M. and De La Cruz, R.B. (2000) Taking part in adolescent sexual health promotion in Peru: community participation from a social psychological perspective, *Journal of Community & Applied Social Psychology*, 10(4), 271–84.

Raphael, D. (2000) Health inequalities in Canada: current discourses and implications for public health action, *Critical Public Health*, 10(2), 193–216.

Renedo, A. and Jovchelovitch, S. (2007) Expert knowledge, cognitive polyphasia and health: a study on social representations of homelessness among professionals working in the voluntary sector in London, *Journal of Health Psychology*, 12(5), 779–90.

Rhodes, R.E., Blanchard, C.M., Matheson, D.H. and Coble, J. (2006) Disentangling motivation, intention, and planning in the physical activity domain, *Psychology of Sport and Exercise*, 7(1), 15–27.

Robertson, A. (1998) Shifting discourses on health in Canada: from health promotion to population health, *Health Promotion International*, 13(2), 155–66.

Robertson, A. and Minkler, M. (1994) New health promotion movement: a critical examination, *Health Education and Behavior*, 21, 295–312.

Rodin, J. and Ickovics, J.R. (1990) Women's health: review and research agenda as we approach the 21st century, *American Psychologist*, 45, 1018–34.

Rogers, M.F. (2003) Review of 'Phenomenology encounters illness: beyond inner states', *Health*, 7(2), 251–5.

Rutter, D. and Quine, L. (eds) (2002) *Changing Health Behaviour*. Buckingham: Open University Press.

Saelens, B.E., Sallis, J.F. and Frank, L.D. (2003) Environmental correlates of walking and cycling: findings from the transportation, urban design, and planning literatures, *Annals of Behavioral Medicine*, 25(2), 80–91.

Saks, M. and Allsop, J. (2007) *Researching Health: Qualitative, Quantitative, and Mixed Methods*. Thousand Oaks, CA: Sage.

Sallis, J.F., Cervero, R.B., Ascher, W. et al. (2006) An ecological approach to creating active living communities, *Annual Review of Public Health*, 27, 297–322.

Sanders, D. and Chopra, M. (2006) Key challenges to achieving health for all in an inequitable society: the case of South Africa, *American Journal of Public Health*, 96(1), 73–8.

Saracci, R. (1997) The World Health Organisation needs to reconsider its definition of health, *British Medical Journal*, 314(7091), 1409.

Sarbin, T.R. (ed.) (1986) *Narrative Psychology: The Storied Nature of Human Conduct.* New York: Praeger.

Sato, L., De Castro Lacaz, F.A. and Bernardo, M.H. (2004) Psychology and the workers' health movement in the state of Sao Paulo (Brazil), *Journal of Health Psychology*, 9(1), 121–30.

Scambler, G. (2002) *Health and Social Change*. Buckingham: Open University Press.

Scambler, G. and Kelleher, D. (2006) New social and health movements: issues of representation and change, *Critical Public Health*, 16(3), 219–31.

Schutz, A. (1967) *The Phenomenology of the Social World*. Evanston: Northwestern University Press.

Schwarzer, R. (2008) Modeling health behavior change: how to predict and modify the adoption and maintenance of health behaviours, *Applied Psychology: An International Review*, 57(1), 1–29.

Seedhouse, D. (1997) *Health Promotion: Philosophy, Prejudice and Practice*. Chichester: John Wiley & Sons.

Seedhouse, D. (1998) *Ethics: The Heart of Health Care*, 2nd edn. Chichester: John Wiley & Sons.

Seeman, T.E. (1996) Social ties and health: the benefits of social integration, *Annals of Epidemiology*, 6(5), 442–51.

Semenza, J.C. and Krishnasamy, P.V. (2007) Design of a health-promoting neighborhood intervention, *Health Promotion Practice*, 8(3), 243–56.

Sheeran, P. and Silverman, M. (2003) Evaluation of three interventions to promote workplace health and safety: evidence for the utility of implementation intentions, *Social Science & Medicine*, 56(10), 2153–63.

Sidell, M. (2003) Older people's health: applying Antonovsky's salutogenic paradigm, in M. Siddell, L. Jones, J. Katz, A. Peberdy and J. Douglas (eds), *Debates and Dilemmas in Promoting Health: A Reader*, 2nd edn. Basingstoke: Palgrave Macmillan.

Silverstone, R. (1999) *Why Study the Media?* London: Sage.

Sims-Schouten, W., Riley, S.C. and Willig, C. (2007) Critical realism in discourse analysis: a presentation of a systematic method of analysis using women's talk of motherhood, childcare and female employment as an example, *Theory & Psychology*, 17(1), 101–24.

Singh-Manoux, A. and Marmot, M. (2005) Role of socialization in explaining social inequalities in health, *Social Science & Medicine*, 60(9), 2129–33.

Smedley, B.D. (2006) Expanding the frame of understanding disparities: from a focus on health systems to social and economic systems, *Health Education and Behavior*, 33(4), 538–41.

Smedley, B., Stith, A.Y. and Nelson, A.R. (eds) (2003) *Unequal Treatment: Confronting Racial and Ethnic Disparities in Health Care*. Washington, DC: The National Academies Press.

Smith, J.A. (2004) Reflecting on the development of interpretative phenomenological analysis and its contribution to qualitative research in psychology, *Qualitative Research in Psychology*, 1, 39–54.

Smith, N.L. and Brandon, P.R. (eds) (2007) *Fundamental Issues in Evaluation*. New York: Guilford Press.

Smith, J.A. and Osborn, M. (2007) Pain as an assault on the self: an interpretative phenomenological analysis of the psychological impact of chronic benign low back pain, *Psychology & Health*, 22(5), 517–34.

Smith, J.A., Jarman, M. and Osborn, M. (1999) Doing interpretive phenomenological analysis, in M. Murray and K. Chamberlain (eds), *Qualitative Health Psychology*. Thousand Oaks, CA: Sage, pp. 218–38.

Sporle, A. (2002) Socio-economic differences in health in Māori, in N. Pearce and L. Ellison-Loschmann (eds), *Explanations of Socio-economic Differences in Health*. Wellington, NZ: Centre for Public Health Research, Massey University.

Sporle, A., Pearce, N. and Davis, P. (2002) Social class differences in Māori and non-Māori aged 15–64 during the last two decades, *New Zealand Medical Journal*, 115, 127–31.

Springett, J. (2003) Issues in participatory evaluation, in M. Minkler and N. Wallerstein (eds), *Community-based Participatory Research for Health*. San Francisco, CA: Jossey-Bass, pp. 263–91.

Stam, H.J. (2000). Theorizing health and illness: functionalism, subjectivity and reflexivity, *Journal of Health Psychology*, 5(3), 273–83.

Stam, H.J. (2004) A sound mind in a sound body: a critical historical analysis of health psychology, in M. Murray (ed.), *Critical Health Psychology*. Basingstoke: Palgrave Macmillan, pp. 15–30.

Stephens, C. (2007) Community as practice: social representations of community and their implications for health promotion, *Journal of Community and Applied Social Psychology*, 17, 103–14.

Stephens, C. (2008) Social capital in its place: using social theory to understand social capital and inequalities in health, *Social Science & Medicine*, 66, 1174–84.

Stephens, C. and Breheny, M. (2007) Menopause and the virtuous woman: the importance of the moral order in accounting for medical decision making, *Health (London)*, 12(1), 7–24.

Stephens, C., Budge, R.C. and Carryer, J. (2002) What is this thing called HRT? Discursive construction of medication in situated practice, *Qualitative Health Research*, 12, 347–59.

Stephens, C., Carryer, J. and Budge, C. (2004) To have or to take: discourse, positioning, and narrative identity in women's accounts of HRT, *Health (London)*, 8, 329–50.

Stephenson, M., Jr. (2007) Developing community leadership through the arts in Southside Virginia: social networks, civic identity and civic change, *Community Development Journal*, 42, 79–96.

Stokols, D. (1992) Establishing and maintaining healthy environments: toward a social ecology of health promotion, *American Psychologist*, 47, 6–22.

Sykes, C.M., Willig, C. and Marks, D.F. (2004) Discourses in the European

Commission's 1996–2000 Health Promotion Programme, *Journal of Health Psychology*, 9(1), 131–41.

Szreter, S. and Woolcock, M. (2004) Health by association? Social capital, social theory, and the political economy of public health, *International Journal of Epidemiology*, 33(4), 650–67.

Tesoriero, F. (2006) Strengthening communities through women's self help groups in South India, *Community Development Journal*, 41, 321–33.

Thompson, B. and Kinne, S. (1999) Social change theory: applications to community health, in N. Bracht (ed.), *Health Promotion at the Community Level, 2: New Advances*. Thousand Oaks, CA: Sage, pp. 29–46.

Thomson, H. and Petticrew, M. (2007) Editorial: housing and health, *British Medical Journal*, 334, 434–5.

Tobias, M. and Yeh, L.C. (2006) Do all ethnic groups in New Zealand exhibit socio-economic mortality gradients? *Australian and New Zealand Journal of Public Health*, 30(4), 343–9.

Townsend, P. and Davidson, N. (1982) *Inequalities in Health: The Black Report*. Harmondsworth: Penguin.

Townsend, P., Davidson, N. and Whitehead, M. (1986) *The Black Report and the Health Divide*. Harmondsworth: Penguin.

Tucker, J., Van Teijlingen, E., Philip, K., Shucksmith, J. and Penney, G. (2006) Health demonstration projects: evaluating a community-based health intervention programme to improve young people's sexual health, *Critical Public Health*, 16(3), 175–89.

Turan, J.M., Say, L., Gungor, A.K., Demarco, R., and Yazgan, S. (2003). Community participation for perinatal health in Istanbul. *Health Promotion International*, 18(1), 25–32.

Uutela, A., Absetz, P., Nissinen, A. et al. (2004) Health psychological theory in promoting population health in Pijt-Hme, Finland: first steps toward a type 2 diabetes prevention study, *Journal of Health Psychology*, 9(1), 73–84.

Van Merode, T., Chhem Dy, B., Kros, S. and Lubek, I. (2006) Antiretrovirals for employees of large companies in Cambodia, *Lancet*, 368(9541), 1065.

Ville, I. and Khlat, M. (2007) Meaning and coherence of self and health: an approach based on narratives of life events, *Social Science & Medicine*, 64(4), 1001–14.

Visser, M.J., Schoeman, J.B. and Perold, J.J. (2004) Evaluation of HIV/AIDS prevention in South African schools, *Journal of Health Psychology*, 9(2), 263–80.

Von Lengerke, T. (2006) Public health is an interdiscipline, and about wholes and parts, *Journal of Health Psychology*, 11(3), 395–9.

Wakefield, S.E.L. and Poland, B. (2005) Family, friend or foe? Critical reflections on the relevance and role of social capital in health promotion and community development, *Social Science & Medicine*, 60(12), 2819–32.

Wallack, L. (2003) The role of media in creating social capital: a new direction for public health, in R. Hofrichter (ed.), *Health and Social Justice: Politics, Ideology, and Inequity in the Distribution of Disease*. San Francisco, CA: Jossey-Bass, pp. 594–626.

Wallerstein, N. (2006) *What is the Evidence on Effectiveness of Empowerment to Improve Health?* Health Evidence Network Report. Copenhagen: WHO Regional Office for Europe. Available at: www.euro.who.int/Document/E88086.pdf (accessed 15 Jan. 2008).

Wallerstein, N. and Duran, B. (2003) The conceptual, historical, and practice roots of community based participatory research and related participatory traditions, in M. Minkler and N. Wallerstein (eds), *Community-based Participatory Research for Health*. San Francisco, CA: Jossey-Bass, pp. 27–52.

Wang, C., Yi, W., Tao, Z. and Carovano, K. (1998) Photovoice as a participatory health promotion strategy, *Health Promotion International*, 13(1), 75–86.

Washer, P. and Joffe, H. (2006) The 'hospital superbug': social representations of MRSA, *Social Science & Medicine*, 63(8), 2141–52.

Waterman, H., Marshall, M., Noble, J. et al. (2007) The role of action research in the investigation and diffusion of innovations in health care: the PRIDE project, *Qualitative Health Research*, 17(3), 373–81.

Webster, C. and French, J. (2003) The cycle of conflict: the history of the public health and health promotion movements, in M. Sidell, L. Jones, J. Katz, A. Peberdy and J. Douglas (eds), *Debates and Dilemmas in Promoting Health*, 2nd edn. Buckingham: Open University Press.

Welch Cline, R.J. and McKenzie, N.J. (1996) Women and AIDS: the lost population, in R.L. Parrott and C.M. Condit (eds), *Evaluating Women's Health Messages*. Thousand Oaks, CA: Sage.

Wells, R., Ford, E.W., McClure, J.A., Holt, M.L. and Ward, A. (2007) Community-based coalitions' capacity for sustainable action: the role of relationships, *Health Education & Behavior*, 34(1), 124–39.

Wendel-Vos, W., Droomers, M., Kremers, S., Brug, J. and Van Lenthe, F. (2007) Potential environmental determinants of physical activity in adults: a systematic review. *Obesity Reviews*, 8(5), 425–40.

Wetherell, M. and Potter, J. (1992) *Mapping the Language of Racism: Discourse and the Legitimation of Exploitation*. New York: Columbia University Press.

Whaley, A.L. (2003) Ethnicity/race, ethics, and epidemiology, *Journal of the National Medical Association*, 95(8), 736–42.

Whitehead, M. (2007) A typology of actions to tackle social inequalities in health, *Journal of Epidemiology and Community Health*, 61(6), 473–8.

Whitehead, K.A., Kriel, A.J. and Richter, L.M. (2005) Barriers to conducting a community mobilization intervention among youth in a rural South African community, *Journal of Community Psychology*, 33(3), 253–9.

Wight, D. and Abraham, C. (2000) From psycho-social theory to sustainable classroon practice: developing a research-based teacher-delivered sex education programme, *Health Education Research*, 15(1), 25–38.

Wight, D., Raab, G.R., Henderson, M. et al. (2002) Limits of teacher delivered sex education: interim behavioural outcomes from randomised trial, *British Medical Journal* (doi:1410.1136/bmj.1324.7351.1430), 324, 1430.

Wilkinson, R.G. (1999) Health, hierarchy, and social anxiety, *Annals of the New York Academy of Sciences*, 896(1), 48–63.

Wilkinson, R.G. (2005). *The Impact of Inequality: How to Make Sick Societies Healthier*. London: Routledge.

Wilkinson, R. and Marmot, M. (eds) (2003) *Social Determinants of Health: The Solid Facts*, 2nd edn. Barcelona: World Health Organization, Europe.

Wilkinson, R. and Marmot, M. (2006) *The Solid Facts: The Social Determinants of Health*. Barcelona: World Health Organization, Europe.

Wilkinson, R.G. and Pickett, K.E. (2006) Income inequality and population health: a review and explanation of the evidence, *Social Science & Medicine*, 62(7), 1768–84.

Williams, G. (1984) The genesis of chronic illness: narrative re-construction, *Sociology of Health & Illness*, 6(2), 175–200.

Williams, G. (1993) Chronic illness and the pursuit of virtue in everyday life, in R. Radley (ed.), *Worlds of Illness: Biographical and Cultural Perspectives on Health and Disease*. London: Routledge, pp. 71–91.

Williams, S.J. (1995) Theorising class, health and lifestyles: can Bourdieu help us? *Sociology of Health and Illness*, 17(5), 577–604.

Williams, S.J. (2003) Beyond meaning, discourse and the empirical world: critical realist reflections on health, *Social Theory and Health*, 1(1), 42–71.

Williams, D.R., Yu, Y. Jackson, J.S. and Anderson, N.B. (1997) Racial differences in physical and mental health: socio-economic status, stress and discrimination, *Journal of Health Psychology*, 2(3), 335–51.

Williams, L., Labonte, R. and O'Brien, M. (2003) Empowering social action through narratives of identity and culture, *Health Promotion International*, 18(1), 33–40.

Willig, C. (1993). Beyond appearances: a critical realist approach to social constructionist work, in J. Cromby and D. Nightingale (eds), *Social Constructionist Psychology: A Critical Analysis of Theory and Practice*. Buckingham: Open University Press.

Willig, C. (ed.) (1999) *Applied Discourse Analysis: Social and Psychological Interventions*. Buckingham: Open University Press.

Willig, C. (2000) A discourse-dynamic approach to the study of subjectivity in health psychology, *Theory and Psychology*, 10, 547–70.

Wilson, N., Dasho, S., Martin, A.C. et al. (2007) Engaging young adolescents in social action through photovoice: the youth empowerment strategies (YES!) project, *The Journal of Early Adolescence*, 27(2), 241–61.

Wimbush, E. and Watson, J. (2000) An evaluation framework for health promotion: theory, quality and effectiveness, *Evaluation*, 6(3), 301–21.

Woodward, A., Crampton, P., Howden-Chapman, P. and Salmond, C. (2000) Poverty – still a health hazard, *New Zealand Medical Journal*, 113(1105), 67–8.

Woolcock, M. (1998) Social capital and economic development: toward a theoretical synthesis and policy framework, *Theory and Society*, 27(2), 151–208.

WHO (World Health Organization) (2002) *The World Health Report 2002: Reducing Risks, Promoting Healthy Life*. Available at: www.who.int/whr/2002/en/index.html (accessed 26 Feb. 2008).

WHO (World Health Organization) (2008) www.who.int/en/ (accessed 7 Feb. 2008).

Yardley, L. (ed.) (1997) *Material Discourses of Health and Illness*. London: Routledge.

Zakus, J. and Lysack, C. (1998) Revisiting community participation, *Health Policy and Planning*, 13(1), 1–12.

Ziersch, A.M. (2005) Health implications of access to social capital: findings from an Australian study, *Social Science & Medicine*, 61(10), 2119–31.

Zoellner, J., Connell, C.L., Santell, R. et al. (2007) Fit for life steps: results of a community walking intervention in the Rural Mississippi Delta, *Progress in Community Health Partnerships: Research, Education, and Action*, 1(1), 49–60.

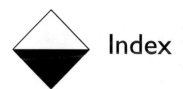

Index

Related books from Open University Press

Purchase from www.openup.co.uk or order through your local bookseller

---

HEALTH COMMUNICATION
Theory and Practice

Dianne Berry

♦ Why is effective communication important in health, and what does this involve?
♦ What issues arise when communicating with particular populations, or in difficult circumstances?
♦ How can the communication skills of health professionals be improved?

Effective health communication is now recognised to be a critical aspect of healthcare at both the individual and wider public level. Good communication is associated with positive health outcomes, whereas poor communication is associated with a number of negative outcomes. This book assesses current research and practice in the area and provides some practical guidance for those involved in communicating health information. It draws on material from several disciplines, including health, medicine, psychology, sociology, linguistics, pharmacy, statistics, and business and management.

The book examines:

♦ The importance of effective communication in health
♦ Basic concepts and processes in communication
♦ Communication theories and models
♦ Communicating with particular groups and in difficult circumstances
♦ Ethical issues
♦ Communicating with the wider public and health promotion
♦ Communication skills training

Health Communication is key reading for students and researchers who need to understand the factors that contribute to effective communication in health, as well as for health professionals who need to communicate effectively with patients and others. It provides a thorough and up to date, evidence-based overview of this important topic, examining the theoretical and practical aspects of health communication for those whose work involves communication with patients, relatives and other carers.

Contents: *Preface – Introduction to health communication – Basic forms of communication – Underlying theories and models – Communication between patients and health professionals – Communicating with particular populations in healthcare – Communication of difficult information and in difficult circumstances – Health promotion and communicating with the wider public – Communication skills training – References – Index.*

2006 152pp   978–0–335–21870–7 (Paperback)   978–0–335–21871–4 (Hardback)

PUBLIC HEALTH
Social Context and Action

Angela Scriven and Sebastian Garman

"From Sure Start to healthy workplaces, health action zones to community regeneration, this volume makes the leap from research to action."
        Professor Richard Parish, Chief Executive, The Royal Society for the Promotion of Health

♦ What is public health and how has it changed over time?
♦ What is the social context of public health and what are the dominant 21st century issues?
♦ What strategies are in place to address population health?

This important book makes a significant contribution to the emergent body of public health knowledge by examining debates around the social context of health, including key socio-economic, environmental and cultural factors. In doing so, the text locates within a social context the theoretical debates and problems surrounding public health, and analyzes the practical public health strategies and solutions that have been developed to address them.

The book moves beyond traditional theoretical discourse to include coverage of:

♦ The thinking, frameworks and processes that are actively shaping public health in the 21st century
♦ Provides tangible examples of public health strategies that have recently been introduced to tackle the social determinants of health
♦ The use of media strategies to promote health

Public Health is key reading for students undertaking courses in health studies, health promotion, nursing, public health, social policy, social work and sociology. In addition to a wide student readership, the book's focus on public health action and current practice also makes it highly relevant to professionals.

The text brings together a distinguished group of practitioners, social scientists and public health experts who contribute their ideas and research.

Contributors: *Amanda Amos, Mel Bartley, Linda Bauld, Hannah Bradby, Tarani Chandola, Jeff Collin, Paul Fleming, Colin Fudge, Sebastian Garman, Ben Gidley, Jenny Head, David Hunter, Martin King, Roderick Lawrence, Kelley Lee, Yaojun Li, Mhairi Mackenzie, Alex Marsh, Antony Morgan, Jennie Popay, Graham Scambler, Sasha Scambler, Angela Scriven, Nick Watson.*

Contents: *List of figures and tables – Notes on contributors – Acknowledgements – Foreword – Public health: An overview of social context and action – Public health: Historical context and current agenda – Part 1: Social context of public health – Trends and transitions: The sociopolitical context of public health – Social patterning of health behaviours – Resilience and change: The relationship of work to health – Social capital, social exclusion and wellbeing – Ethnicity and racism in the politics of health – Disability and public health: From resistance to empowerment – Mass media, lifestyle and public health – Globalisation and public health – Part 2: Public health action – Healthy public policies: Rhetoric or effective reality? – Health action zones: Multi agency partnerships to improve health – Sure Start: An upstream approach to reducing health inequalities – Community participation for health: Reducing health inequalities and building social capital? – Workplaces as settings for public health development – Healthy Cities: Key principles for professional practice – From self regulation to legislation: The social impact of public health action on smoking – Housing, health and wellbeing: A public health action priority – Author index – Subject index.*

2007 256pp   978–0–335–22150–9 (Paperback) 978–0–335–22151–6 (Hardback)

UNEQUAL LIVES
Health and Socioeconomic Inequalities

Hilary Graham

"With the compelling evidence that more redistributive universal welfare benefits and education provide the main escalator to reducing inequalities, this is a timely and thought-provoking book for all those concerned to reduce our societies' embedded structural inequalities, cumulative disadvantages and health inequalities."

Australian and New Zealand Journal of Public Health

"Unequal Lives is the book that we have all been waiting for. In this skilfully crafted volume, Hilary Graham makes the vital connection between health inequalities and social inequalities in a way that opens up new understandings of both concepts and consequences for policy. Scholarly yet accessible, this is a 'must read' book for researchers, policymakers and practitioners alike."

Margaret Whitehead, WH Duncan Professor of Public Health, University of Liverpool, UK

♦ What is meant by health inequalities and socioeconomic inequalities?
♦ What evidence is there to support the link between socioeconomic status and health?
♦ Why do these links persist over time, between and within societies, and across people's lives?
♦ What part do policies play in the persistence of social and health inequalities?

Unequal Lives provides an evidence-based introduction to social and health inequalities. It brings together research from social epidemiology, sociology and social policy to guide the reader to an understanding of why people's lives and people's health remain so unequal, even in rich societies where there is more than enough for all.

The book introduces the non-specialist to key concepts like health inequalities and health inequities, social class and socioeconomic position, social determinants and life course, as well as to the key indicators of health and socioeconomic position.

It provides a wealth of evidence on socioeconomic inequalities in health at both national and global level, and explores how these inequalities persist as countries industrialise, patterns of employment and family life change, and chronic diseases emerge as the big killers.

Consideration is given to policy and its impact on inequalities within the UK, Europe and beyond and an assessment made of health inequalities throughout the life.

This new book from best selling author Hilary Graham is of particular interest to students in sociology, social policy, health studies, health promotion and public health as well as to social work and community nursing students and those working in the health and welfare fields.

Contents: *Acknowledgements – Introduction – Part 1: Key terms – Health inequalities and inequities – Measures of health and health inequalities – Socioeconomic inequalities – Measures of socioeconomic position – Part 2: Patterns of unequal health – Health inequalities: Global, national and historical – Health inequalities across changes in disease – Part 3: Understandings – Social determinants of health and health inequalities – Socioeconomic inequalities across generations: Occupation and education – Socioeconomic inequalities across generations: Partnership and parenthood – Health across unequal lives – Unequal lives: Policy matters – Concluding comment – Bibliography.*

2007 260pp   978–0–335–21369–6 (Paperback) 978–0–335–21370–2 (Hardback)

HEALTH PROMOTION PRACTICE
Building Empowered Communities

Glenn Laverack

"The book provides an excellent combination of broad theoretical background with a generous helping of vocational guidance on the practice of health promotion."

scotregen

"A very welcome addition to the practical side of health promotion! Laverack's brief and simply-worded text weaves together just the right balance of theory, evidence, tips and case studies to satisfy the new learner looking to gain a grasp of health promotion's empowering whole, while still offering new insights to the more seasoned practitioner."

Ronald Labonté, *Institute of Population Health, University of Ottawa*

♦ How can health promotion practitioners help communities to become more empowered?
♦ How do you encourage different communities to work together towards a shared goal?
♦ How can you focus your resources to be most effective in building empowered communities?
♦ How do you evaluate your success (and failures) in building empowered communities?

Power and empowerment are two complex concepts that are central to health promotion practice. People experience empowerment in many different ways and this book explains an approach that has been used by health promoters to intentionally build and evaluate empowerment. The book provides a special focus on communities and is illustrated throughout with useful field experiences in the United Kingdom, Asia, North America, the Pacific region and Africa.

The book aims to provide the reader with:

♦ An understanding of the key concepts of power and empowerment and the link to improved health outcomes in the context of health promotion programmes
♦ An understanding of practical approaches that can be used in health promotion programming to build and evaluate empowered communities
♦ Case study examples of how communities can be empowered in practice

This unique book offers sound theoretical principles to underpin the practical approaches used to build empowered communities and brings together new and innovative approaches in health promotion practice.

Health Promotion Practice is essential reading for health promotion students and practitioners who want to learn more about innovative approaches to build empowered communities in their every-day work. It will inspire them to work in more empowering ways in health promotion practice and to carefully contemplate how they can influence the way others gain power.

Contents: *Preface – An overview of the book – Health promotion practice – Communities and community based interaction – Health and empowerment – Empowerment & health promotion programming – 'Unpacking' community empowerment for strategic planning – Evaluating community empowerment – Empowerment in action: An issues based approach – Empowerment in action: A community-based approach – Building empowered communities in health promotion practice – Index – Bibliography.*

2007 168pp   978–0–335–22057–1 (Paperback) 978–0–335–22058–8 (Hardback)

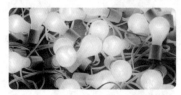
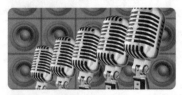
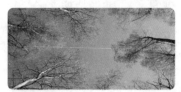
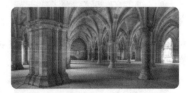
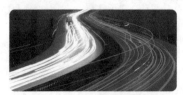
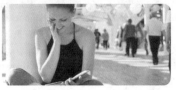
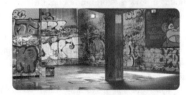
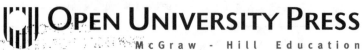